GIS Automated Delineation of Hospital Service Areas

GIS Automated Delineation of Hospital Service Areas

Fahui Wang and Changzhen Wang

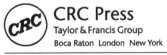

CRC Press
Taylor & Francis Group
Boca Raton London New York

CRC Press is an imprint of the
Taylor & Francis Group, an **informa** business

For computer programs, sample data sets, and user manuals, please visit the authors' website at faculty.lsu.edu/Fahui

First edition published 2022
by CRC Press
6000 Broken Sound Parkway NW, Suite 300, Boca Raton, FL 33487-2742

and by CRC Press
2 Park Square, Milton Park, Abingdon, Oxon, OX14 4RN

© 2022 Taylor & Francis Group, LLC

CRC Press is an imprint of Taylor & Francis Group, LLC

Library of Congress Cataloging-in-Publication Data
Names: Wang, Fahui, 1967– author. | Wang, Changzhen, author.
Title: GIS automated delineation of hospital service areas / Fahui Wang and Changzhen Wang.
Description: First edition. | Boca Raton : CRC Press, 2022. |
Includes bibliographical references and index.
Identifiers: LCCN 2021027194 | ISBN 9780367202286 (hardback) |
ISBN 9781032079493 (paperback) | ISBN 9780429260285 (ebook)
Subjects: LCSH: Health facilities—Location—Data processing. |
Hospital care—Geographic information systems. | Hospital care—Data processing. |
Hospital utilization—Geographic information systems. |
Hospital utilization—Data processing. | Health planning—Geographic information systems. | Health planning—Data processing.
Classification: LCC RA967.7 .W36 2022 | DDC 362.110285—dc23
LC record available at https://lccn.loc.gov/2021027194

ISBN: 9780367202286 (hbk)
ISBN: 9781032079493 (pbk)
ISBN: 9780429260285 (ebk)

DOI: 10.1201/9780429260285

Typeset in Palatino
by codeMantra

Contents

Foreword ix
Preface xi
Authors xiii
List of Major GIS Datasets and Program Files xv

1. Why Hospital Service Areas? 1
   1.1   Hospital Service Area (HSA) as a Functional Region 1
   1.2   Value of HSAs 2
   1.3   Study Area and Data 4
   1.4   Overview of Remaining Chapters 7

2. Estimating Distance and Travel Time Matrices in GIS 11
   2.1   Measures of Distance and Travel Time 11
   2.2   Computing Distance and Drive Time Matrices in
         ArcGIS Pro 13
         2.2.1   Computing Euclidean and Geodesic Distance
                 Matrices in ArcGIS Pro 14
         2.2.2   Computing a Drive Time Matrix in ArcGIS Pro 15
   2.3   Estimating a Transit Travel Time Matrix in ArcGIS Pro 19
   2.4   Estimating Drive Time and Transit Time Matrices
         by Google Maps API 25
   2.5   Estimating a Large Drive Time Matrix by a Differential
         Sampling Approach 32
         2.5.1   Estimating Preliminary Inter-zonal Times 33
         2.5.2   Calibrating Inter-zonal Times on Randomly
                 Sampled OD Pairs by Google Maps API 34
         2.5.3   Appending Intra-zonal Times 35
   2.6   Summary 37

3. Analysis of Spatial Behavior of Health Care Utilization in
   Distance Decay 39
   3.1   Distance Decay Functions 40
   3.2   Value of Analyzing Distance Decay Effects in Health Care
         Studies 41
   3.3   Deriving the Distance Decay Functions by the Spatial
         Interaction Model 44
         3.3.1   Estimating the Spatial Interaction Model 44
         3.3.2   Distance Decay Effects across Geographic Areas in
                 Florida 47

3.4   Deriving the Distance Decay Functions by a
        Complementary Cumulative Distribution Curve 53
        3.4.1   Estimating the Complementary
                 Cumulative Distribution Function 53
        3.4.2   Distance Decay Effects Across Population
                 Groups in Florida 54
3.5   Summary 59

4. Delineating Hospital Service Areas by the Dartmouth Method 61
4.1   History and Applications of Dartmouth HSAs and HRRs 61
4.2   The Dartmouth Method for Defining HSAs and HRRs 63
        4.2.1   Defining HSAs by the Refined Dartmouth Method 63
        4.2.2   Defining HRRs by the Refined Dartmouth Method 67
4.3   Automating the Refined Dartmouth Method for HSA &
        HRR Delineations 69
4.4   Delineating HSAs and HRRs in Florida by the Refined
        Dartmouth Method 77
        4.4.1   Delineating HSAs and HRRs in Florida by the
                 Automated Toolkit 77
        4.4.2   Calculating Indices for 1993 Dartmouth HSAs and
                 HRRs in Florida by the Toolkit 82
        4.4.3   Evaluating HSAs and HRRs by the Refined
                 Dartmouth Method 85
4.5   Summary 90

5. Delineating Hospital Service Areas by the Huff Model 93
5.1   The Proximal Area Method and Its Implementation in GIS 94
        5.1.1   Defining Proximal Areas in Euclidean
                 Distance in GIS 94
        5.1.2   Defining Proximal Areas in Travel Time in GIS 97
5.2   The Huff Model and Extensions 101
        5.2.1   From Reilly's Law to the Huff Model 101
        5.2.2   Extensions to the Huff Model 103
5.3   Implementing the Huff Model for Delineating HSAs in
        ArcGIS Pro 104
5.4   Automated Delineation of HSAs by Integrating the Huff
        Model and Dartmouth Method 111
5.5   Summary 119

**6. Delineating Hospital Service Areas by Network Community
Detection Methods** 121
6.1   Community Detection Methods: From Louvain to Leiden 122
6.2   Spatially Constrained Louvain and Leiden Methods 125

6.3   Automated Delineation of HSAs and HRRs and a Case
Study in Florida.. 129
    6.3.1   Automating the ScLouvain and ScLeiden
Methods in ArcGIS Pro... 129
    6.3.2   Delineating HSAs and HRRs in Florida by the
ScLouvain and ScLeiden Methods 131
    6.3.3   Computational Performances of the
ScLouvain and ScLeiden Methods 136
6.4   Comparing HSAs and HRRs by ScLouvain, ScLeiden, and
Refined Dartmouth Methods 139
6.5   Summary.. 150

7. **Delineating Cancer Service Areas in the
Northeast Region of the USA**.. 153
7.1   Study Area and Cancer Care Data 154
7.2   Interpolating Suppressed Service Volumes 155
7.3   Delineating CSAs by ScLouvain and ScLeiden in the
Northeast Region 158
7.4   Variation of Distance Decay Behavior across
CSAs in the Northeast Region.. 163
7.5   Summary.. 170

**Appendix A: User Guide: Estimating a Large OD
Drive Time Matrix** 173

**Appendix B: User Guide: How to Create Curved-Line and
Straight-Line Network Flow Maps** 187

References 197

Index... 203

Foreword

Ralph Waldo Emerson counselled that we should "not go where the path may lead, go instead where there is no path and leave a trail". This is exactly what Dr. Fahui Wang has done with his intellectual pursuits over the years that I have known him. He has left a trail of innovative methods for deriving health services areas in ways that both reflect the complex reality of health care delivery and provide accessible tools for a variety of stakeholders. I first knew of Dr. Wang as I was earning my PhD many years ago. By the time I was a tenured professor at Dartmouth's Geisel School of Medicine, my icon in the field of geospatial methods for healthcare was my collaborator and friend. I have been a cancer health services researcher, who also has degrees in geography and health informatics, for my entire career. Now, as Senior Director for Population Sciences, Professor of Population Health Sciences, and Huntsman Cancer Institute Presidential Endowed Chair in Cancer Research, with decades of funding from the National Institutes of Health under my proverbial belt, and almost 200 published papers, I know the field of healthcare delivery well. I also know that collaborating with brilliant people outside of my field is the best way to make an impact with one's research. What a highlight of my career that one of these brilliant people is Dr. Fahui Wang! Dr. Wang and I have co-led National Cancer Institute-funded work, published many papers together, and have co-mentored graduate students.

Much of what I've learned from Dr. Wang is covered in this book—which is at least true from a scientific perspective; there is so much more from a human perspective that I have learned—hence my unbounded respect for him as a person. Readers of this book will not have the benefit of the latter as I have, but *will* gain an understanding of the most advanced, sophisticated, and applicable geospatial methods for measuring and evaluating health-care delivery from a large-scale, population-based perspective. Readers will understand the origins of health service areas, *what* they are, *why* they matter, the dominant methods for *how* they are derived, *when* particular methods are most applicable, and *who* can use them (spoiler alert!—the answer is: anyone who reads this book, digests it, and chooses to apply the tools covered in this book that have been made publicly available by Dr. Wang and his co-author Ms. Changzhen Wang). The beauty of this book is that it takes very sophisticated, state-of-the-art methods, developed and/or adapted by them, explicates those as can be found nowhere else, and then shares the GIS-automated methods they developed in efficient, user-friendly customized tools.

Dr. Fahui Wang has written and edited several other books, but this one stands out as the only one of its kind in the intersecting fields of geography and health services research. That is very fitting, as Dr. Fahui Wang is internationally renowned for his groundbreaking work in spatially integrated social sciences, public policy, and planning—a true interdisciplinary scholar, creative intellectual, technical guru, and translator of advanced methods in usable applications. Readers of this book have the incredible opportunity to benefit from Dr. Fahui Wang's expertise, as I have been so fortunate to do over the past 8 years of my career working with him. As a nationally recognized researcher in the field of cancer care delivery, I *know* the tremendous importance of this book's contributions to the field, and the impact of its innovations in geospatial methods. I urge readers to extend this impact to your own areas/fields of research or policy, as is made eminently possible to you through this book.

Tracy Onega, PhD, MS, MA, MPAS

Huntsman Cancer Institute Presidential Endowed
Chair in Cancer Research
Senior Director, Population Sciences
Professor, Department of Population
Health Sciences, University of Utah
Huntsman Cancer Institute
Salt Lake City, Utah

Preface

My interest in hospital service areas (HSAs) started from a conversation with Dr. Imam Xierali about a decade ago. At the time, as the Manager for Public Health and Diversity Initiatives at the Association of American Medical Colleges (AAMC) in Washington, DC, he was vastly aware of major issues in public health. He raised the issue of HSAs and its value in public health studies and policy and sought my perspective as our interests overlap in GIS health. I was instantly convinced that it would be a fruitful pursuit to develop GIS methods for HSA delineation and related applications.

We went on to co-advise Peng Jia, a PhD student, who was searching for a dissertation topic in health geography in 2013. With the 2011 Healthcare Cost and Utilization Project (HCUP) data in Florida provided by Imam, it made a lot of sense for Peng to work on the project of delineating HSAs and hospital referral regions (HRRs) in Florida. Peng was a quick learner, and we struck gold quickly with our first co-authored paper on the topic winning the 2015 HCUP Outstanding Article of the Year Award (Policy Winner) from the Agency for Healthcare Research and Quality, U.S. Department of Health and Human Services (Jia et al., 2015). After that, we co-authored four more articles on Huff-model-based HSA delineation, HRR delineation, HSA–HRR hierarchical construction, and variations in distance decay effects in inpatient care. Another PhD student of mine, Yujie Hu, was also interested in the issue, and I guided him to explore the network community detection approach in advancing the work of HSA delineation. The result was reported in another paper (Hu et al., 2018). All have become important foundations for this book.

I have also benefited a great deal from the friendship and collaborations with Dr. Tracy Onega, a renowned cancer epidemiologist and health services researcher. Tracy was intimately knowledgeable of the Dartmouth Atlas of Health Care Project since her graduate student years there and went on to become a professor in the Geisel School of Medicine at Dartmouth. Naturally she has a keen interest in HSAs, the very concept piloted by the Dartmouth Atlas of Health Care Project. In 2017, we were awarded a National Institute of Cancer (NCI) grant to develop automated GIS methods for defining cancer service areas (CSAs) in the USA. My new PhD student Changzhen Wang, with a strong background in GIS software engineering, instantly became a reliable source of assistance on the project since she joined our program in 2018. She led the development of a set of automated tools in ArcGIS Pro for delineating CSAs, and the methodology is equally applicable for HSAs. Tracy, Changzhen, and I have co-authored several journal articles to report some preliminary findings from this funded project, and further advanced the earlier work on HSAs. I am so grateful to Tracy, now in the Huntsman Cancer Institute of University of Utah, for writing the Foreword.

It was a natural and wise decision for me to extend my invitation to Changzhen as a co-author of the book. She graciously accepted it and has been a dream collaborator on this endeavor. Not only has she taken on most of the heavy lifting tasks (e.g., programming, implementing case studies and related writing, designing graphics and maps), but she has also suggested several initiatives and followed through with them expeditiously. By working closely with each other, we have largely met our targeted deadlines for each chapter and ensured the overall quality in our writings and associated computer programs.

This book intends to mainly serve upper-level undergraduate and graduate students, researchers, and professionals in *geography, public health, urban and regional planning,* and related fields. It provides the best practice and a one-stop solution for a popular task, delineation of hospital service areas. The methods can be applied to similar tasks of defining any functional regions such as trade area in market analysis, catchment area for a service, and hinterlands in a system of cities. A Web site under my LSU faculty page (faculty.lsu.edu/fahui) will be developed and maintained by the authors to disseminate and update computer programs, sample data, and user manuals.

Thanks to Irma Britton, acquisition editor at CRC Press, with whom I have enjoyed a friendship for more than 15 years. Together we pushed three books through the arduous publication process at CRC Press before this one: (1) *Quantitative Methods and Applications in GIS* (2006), (2) *Quantitative Methods and Socioeconomic Applications in GIS* (2nd edition) (2015), and (3) *GIS-based Simulation and Analysis of Intra-urban Commuting* (2019, with Yujie Hu as the primary author). She encouraged me to pursue this book project and convinced me to sign a contract in 2018.

As soon as I was freed from my administrative duty in the early summer of 2020, I started working on the book with full efforts. The work continued throughout my sabbatical in the fall 2020 and most of this spring semester. The past year has been challenging for everyone including myself and our family. I had planned some trips on my sabbatical for data collection related to new case studies for the book, and had to call them off. Casualties from those cancelled trips included a couple of chapters in the original book proposal. I also experienced various challenges while working from home. At the same time, the commitment to finishing the book under contract has helped me concentrate better. Research for the book and the writing have almost become therapeutic for me.

As I wrap up the Preface to cap this memorable journey, tomorrow will come, and I will be ready to receive my second COVID-19 vaccination shot.

On behalf of my co-author Changzhen, we dedicate the book to all health care workers who have worked tirelessly during this difficult time!

Fahui Wang
Baton Rouge

For computer programs, sample data sets, and user manuals, please visit the authors' website at faculty.lsu.edu/Fahui

Authors

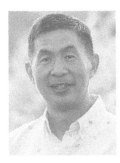

Fahui Wang, PhD, is Cyril & Tutta Vetter Alumni Professor in the Department of Geography and Anthropology, Louisiana State University. He earned a BS degree in geography from Peking University, China, an MA degree in economics, and a PhD degree in city and regional planning from The Ohio State University. His research interests cover human geography (urban, economic, and transportation), city and regional planning, crime analysis, and public health, with a methodological focus in spatial analytics in GIS. According to Scopus 2020, he is among the top 1% most-cited researchers in Geography in the world.

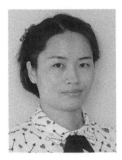

Changzhen Wang is a PhD candidate of geography in the Department of Geography and Anthropology, Louisiana State University. She earned a BS degree from Southwest Jiaotong University and MEng degree from Wuhan University, both in GIS, in China. Her research focuses on development and applications of GIS, computational methods, network analysis, and geo-visualization in public health, urban studies, and transportation.

List of Major GIS Datasets and Program Files

The Florida folder contains all data, produced results, and program tools:

1. FL _ HSA.gdb: a GIS geodatabase that contains feature classes and tables used in Chapters 1–6 and Appendix B.

2. FL _ Ntwk.gdb: a GIS geodatabase that contains a road network dataset and a transit network dataset (as a result) to estimate drive time and transit time in Chapter 2 and define proximal areas in Chapter 5.

3. FL _ MDT _ PublicTransit: a subfolder that contains txt files used for public transit time estimation in Chapter 2.

4. TransitNetworkTemplate.xml: a template used to create transit network dataset in Chapter 2.

5. AddGTFStoND _ UsersGuide.html: a user guide for estimating transit time for ArcMap users in Chapter 2.

6. ODFlowData: a subfolder that contains a node file, an edge file, and Gephi software to create a curved-line network flow map in Appendix B.

7. FLplgnAdjAppend.csv: an appended spatial adjacency matrix that accounts for physical connections between ZIP code areas in the study area. This file is used to adjust the spatial adjacency matrix generated from the tool in ArcGIS Pro in Chapters 4 and 6.

8. Reg _ fitfunction.R and Reg _ fitfunction.SAS: R and SAS programs to implement log-transformed regression analysis of five distance decay functions by spatial interaction model (Sub-section 3.3.1 of Chapter 3).

9. Reg _ ccdf.R: an R program to implement regression analysis of five distance decay functions by complementary cumulative distribution curve (Sub-section 3.4.1 of Chapter 3).

10. OD _ All _ Flows.dbf: a DBF file that contains 37,180 records with four variables POPU, NUMBEDS, AllFlows, and Total _ Time for regression analysis programs Reg _ fitfunction.R, Reg _ fitfunction.SAS, or Reg _ ccdf.R as listed above.

11. requirements.txt: Python packages to be installed for the toolkit of "HSA Delineation Pro.tbx" in Chapters 4, 5, and 6.

12. `Google API Pro.tbx`: an ArcGIS toolkit that contains one tool to implement the drive or transit time estimation by Google Maps API in Chapter 2. The required Python script is saved in subfolder `Scripts`.

13. `Huff Model Pro.tbx`: an ArcGIS toolkit that contains two tools to implement the Huff model in Chapter 5: (1) Huff model based on Euclidean or geodesic distance; (2) Huff model based on an external distance table defined by users. The required Python scripts are saved in subfolder `Scripts`.

14. `HSA Delineation Pro.tbx`: an ArcGIS toolkit that contains five tools in Chapters 4, 5, and 6: (1) build a spatial adjacency matrix from a polygon layer; (2) consolidate flows between areas at a finer level (i.e., ZIP codes, census tracts) to flows between areas at a coarser level (e.g., HSAs); (3) delineate HSAs and HRRs by the refined Dartmouth method; (4) calculate some common indices for assessing regionalization outcomes; (5) delineate HSAs and HRRs by the ScLouvain and ScLeiden methods. The required Python scripts are saved in subfolder `Scripts`.

15. `Scripts`: a subfolder that contains all required Python scripts used for ArcGIS toolkits.

16. `Results`: a subfolder that contains results produced in all Chapters and Appendix B.

1

Why Hospital Service Areas?

When a rural hospital is closed (seemingly a national trend in the USA), what will be the impacts on its local residents as well as other hospitals in the region? Has a National Cancer Institute (NCI) Cancer Center been serving the population representative of various demographic groups in its projected catchment area, as required by the federal guidelines? How should Medicare/Medicaid adjust the reimbursement prices for procedures that pertain to local health care markets and over time? Answering all these questions relies on a data-driven, evidence-based, and timely delineation of hospital service areas (HSAs).

1.1 Hospital Service Area (HSA) as a Functional Region

Hospital service areas (HSAs) were pioneered by the Dartmouth Atlas of Health Care Project (http://www.dartmouthatlas.org/). An HSA is an area within which patients receive most of their hospital care and thus captures a local pattern of hospitalization. HSAs are more meaningful analysis units for studies of health care than geopolitical units (e.g., county, state), administrative units (e.g., township, city), or census units (e.g., metropolitan statistical area) because they represent health care markets.

Hospital referral regions (HRRs) are other units developed by the Dartmouth Atlas of Health Care Project and represent regional health care markets anchored by at least one hospital that provides more specialized care such as major cardiovascular surgery procedures and neurosurgery. An HRR is aggregated from HSAs and is thus a larger unit at a coarser geographic scale than HSA for studies of health care utilization, outcomes, and cost. Currently, there are 3,436 Dartmouth HSAs and only 306 Dartmouth HRRs in the USA. According to the *central place theory* (Christaller, 1966), an HRR is a higher-level tertiary hospital market area characterized by higher-order medical services that are available in their anchoring hospital(s) but absent in those anchoring HSAs.

The Dartmouth Atlas of Health Care Project has also developed other health care service areas such as *pediatric surgical areas (PSAs)* (Dartmouth Atlas of Health Care, 2013) and *primary care service areas (PCSAs)* (Goodman et al., 2003) for their respective medical services. Conceivably, for analysis of

DOI: 10.1201/9780429260285-1

any health care service, one needs to define a service area pertaining to that type of service in order to capture its unique market structure. For example, *cancer service areas (CSAs)* are defined for cancer care (Wang et al., 2020). In this book, the term HSA, unless specified or implied otherwise in a context, refers to broadly defined hospital (or health care in general) service area regardless of the service types provided by hospitals or other medical facilities.

In geography, HSA is a type of functional region. A *functional region* is an area around a node, facility, or hub connected by a certain function (e.g., retail distribution, advertisement for a media company, and telecom coverage). Delineation of functional regions occurs by defining regions that are coherent in terms of connections between supply and demand for a service. By defining a functional region, a distinctive market area has a geographic boundary that encompasses many smaller areas more closely connected with the central node(s) than beyond.

The literature in various fields uses other terms that possess the same or similar properties as a functional region. For example, *catchment area (CA)* refers to an area around a facility where most of its clients, patients, or patrons reside. Similarly, *trade area* is "the geographic area from which a store draws most of its customers and within which market penetration is highest" (Ghosh and McLafferty, 1987, p.62). In urban and regional studies, *hinterland* (Wang, 2001) or *urban sphere of influence* (Berry and Lamb, 1974) includes the rural area that maintains the highest volume of commerce, service, and other connections with and around a city.

Defining functional regions is a classic task in geography. It can be as straightforward as assigning areas to their nearest facility to form a proximal region around it, or as complex as untangling a massive interconnected network of interactions. The development of geographic information systems (GIS) has helped advance related methodology, especially in automating the delineation process, spatializing network methods, and visualizing the results. The book focuses on the methods for defining HSAs. While the methods introduced in this book are illustrated in case studies of medical services, they can be applied to delineation of any functional regions.

1.2 Value of HSAs

The purpose of delineating HSAs is to define a reliable unit of analysis for examining the geographic variation of the health care system (Kilaru et al., 2015). Obviously, the definition and choice of an areal unit of analysis affects the validity of findings based on data aggregated in such a unit, commonly known as the *modifiable areal unit problem (MAUP)* (Fotheringham and Wong, 1991). If the unit does not capture the actual health care market structure, corresponding policy and planning strategy would be ill-informed. Here some exemplary studies are cited to illustrate the values of HSAs for designing research, informing health policy, and planning resources.

Glover (1938) is believed to be the first to study geographic variation in health care that helped explain the variation of tonsillectomy rates in Great Britain (Onega et al., 2014). In the USA, Wennberg and Gittelsohn (1973) were among the first to examine the study of geographic variations in health care resource, utilization, and expenditures across small areas in Vermont. However, researchers have long debated about the magnitude and underlying causes of variation. A report by Goodman et al. (2010) revealed that the quality of end-of-life cancer care for Medicare beneficiaries varied significantly across hospitals and the aforementioned Dartmouth HRRs. It helped identify hospitals and geographic regions that aggressively treated those patients with likely unwarranted curative attempts and incurred excessive costs without improving the quality of their last weeks and months. The report has been instrumental in guiding improvements in the development and delivery of symptom control and other palliative care for terminally ill cancer patients.

An influential study reported by the Institute of Medicine (IOM, 2013) also found substantial geographic variations in health care spending in the USA, and such variations were not necessarily associated with quality of care, by largely relying on the same analysis unit Dartmouth HRRs. While the subtitle of the report, "Target Decision-makers, Not Geography", might appear to cast doubt on the promise of geographic and regional efforts to improve US health care services, one major policy recommendation made by the report was to promote the transition to value-based payment models by providing financial incentives for health care providers to reduce costs and improve quality. However, the variability of cost efficiency in individual providers is embedded in the geographic variation across regions. Regional initiatives are just as important as providers-targeted incentives to improve both health and health care (Fisher and Skinner, 2013).

Health care markets also evolve over time as people move, some hospitals close and others open, and transportation networks connecting people and hospitals change. Units such as the Dartmouth HSAs and HRRs defined in the early 1990s have become outdated (Jia et al., 2015, 2020). Hospital closures have left some Dartmouth HSAs without any hospitals, and these units would no longer be suitable for analysis decades later. But many studies still used the same units "in order to preserve the continuity of the database" (Dartmouth Atlas of Health Care, 2011, p.4)[1]. These units need to be updated with more recent data and defined with the methods that better reflect the scientific advancement in the field of deriving functional regions.

---

[1] Per conversations with Dr. Anna N. A. Tosteson and Dr. Jonathan Skinner of the Dartmouth Institute for Health Policy & Clinical Practice on March 23, 2021, the Dartmouth HSAs and HRRs are updated to the current ZIP code areas every year, but their basic geographic boundaries have not changed in order to facilitate longitude studies.

Most recently, the National Cancer Institute (NCI) mandated its designated cancer centers to identify and describe their CAs and document work that specifically addresses the cancer burden, risk factors, incidence, morbidity, mortality, and inequities, within the CAs (Paskett and Hiatt, 2018). While the mandate came without specific guidelines for defining the boundary of CA, its description suggests that CA should capture where a center's patients come from, its marketing area, and where its research participants live. All are important elements for defining an HSA. Defining the CAs for the more than 70 NCI-designated cancer centers consistently is critical to assess whether these hospitals funded by federal resources serve their corresponding population base. This is especially challenging for hospitals without the personnel with highly specialized expertise in GIS and spatial analysis. Delineation of CAs is also important for accurately assessing epidemiological disease burdens and planning health care delivery accordingly (Alegana et al., 2020).

In short, HSAs have increasingly been adopted as a basic geographic unit for health care delivery assessment, management, and planning. The unit needs to pertain to the specific medical service being investigated and be defined in a timely fashion and at a scale suitable for the purpose of research and public policy relevance. Given the increasing volume of data required and complexity of algorithms, it is critical to develop methods that are computationally efficient, adaptable for various scales (from a local region to as large as a nationwide market), and automated without a steep learning curve for public health professionals.

This book sets out to meet these challenges by developing GIS-automated methods that cater to data needs (or lack of some data) and are efficient and easy to use in customized tools.

1.3 Study Area and Data

Unless specified otherwise, the same dataset for one study area is used throughout the book to illustrate various methods.

The study area is the state of Florida. Florida is only contiguously connected with two states—Alabama and Georgia—to the north, and bordered by Gulf of Mexico to the west, Atlantic Ocean to the east, and Straits of Florida to the south. This unique geography makes Florida an ideal study area as the edge effect is limited. *Edge effect* refers to cross-border interactions (e.g., residents in Florida seek health care outside of the state, and residents in other states are cared by hospitals and clinics in the state) which would bias a study if not properly accounted for.

The major data source is the *State Inpatient Database (SID)* of Florida 2011 from the Healthcare Cost and Utilization Project (HCUP) sponsored by the Agency for Healthcare Research and Quality (AHRQ, 2011). The SID includes individual inpatient discharge records in terms of all patients, regardless of payer, from community hospitals in Florida in 2011. It contains variables such as principal and secondary diagnoses and procedures, payment source (e.g., Medicare, Medicaid, and private insurance), total charges, patient ZIP codes, and a unique hospital identifier (http://www.hcup-us. ahrq.gov/sidoverview.jsp). The data are linked with the 2013 American Hospital Association (AHA) survey based on the unique hospital identifier and appended with hospital information such as hospital address, bed size, and hospital type. The Florida 2011 SID consists of inpatient discharge records from all hospitals, including hospital transfers. For patients admitted to multiple hospitals or one patient with multiple admissions, each admission is regarded as a separate record in this analysis. Records associated with hospitals that cannot be identified and records without residence ZIP codes are excluded. The resulting dataset includes 2,392,066 all-payer records (over 90% of the original records).

These individual records are further consolidated to the ZIP code area level for various case studies in this book. This applies to data by patient residential locations (origins), hospitals (destinations), and the OD (origin–destination) flows between them. ZIP code area is the finest spatial resolution for patients in the HCUP data. We have also consolidated hospitals to ZIP code areas and then the OD flow data between them. As discussed in Chapters 4–6, HSAs in the USA are constructed from ZIP code areas since most medical records are geocoded to ZIP code areas. Therefore, it is beneficial to aggregate individual hospital data to ZIP code areas so that the patient service flow network is unified as a spatial network between nodes of ZIP code areas. Furthermore, the aggregation also helps mask data privacy associated with the HCUP data.

Specifically, if a ZIP code area contains multiple hospitals, these hospitals are represented by one single point with the location defined as their weighted mean center and the capacity as their total bed size. In effect, 268 hospitals are consolidated to 213 total hospital ZIP code points; similarly, 197 specialized hospitals (a subset of the 268 hospitals) are consolidated to 192 specialized hospital ZIP code points, hereafter simply referred to as "hospitals" and "specialized hospitals", respectively. Specialized hospitals are those providing cardiovascular surgeries and neurosurgeries and will be used for delineating HRRs. The patient flow volumes are also aggregated to OD flows between ZIP code areas.

A GIS geodatabase FL _ HSA.gdb contains the following data:

1. A polygon feature class ZIP _ Code _ Area includes 983 ZIP code areas with demand defined in field POPU for population in 2010, and its corresponding point feature class is ZIP _ Points. The total population in the study area is 18,803,233.

2. A point feature class Hosp _ ZIP includes 213 "hospitals" (unique ZIP code points) with capacity defined in field NUMBEDS for staffed bed size.

3. A point feature class SPHosp _ ZIP includes 192 "specialized hospitals" (unique ZIP code points) with capacity defined in field SPNUMBEDS for staffed bed size.

4. A stand-alone table OD _ All _ Flows includes 209,379 (=983*213) records with field Total _ Time _ min for travel time in minutes from each unique residential ZIP code area to each unique hospital ZIP code area and field AllFlows for corresponding volumes of all patient service flows between ZIP code areas. It has 37,180 non-zero flows (i.e., the number of records with AllFlows>0). The total service volume (i.e., the sum of AllFlows) is 2,392,066.

5. A stand-alone table OD _ CardNeur _ Flows includes 14,168 records with field CardNeurFlows for volumes of cardiovascular surgery and neurosurgery patient service flows from each unique residential ZIP code area to each unique specialized hospital ZIP code area. The total volume (i.e., the sum of CardNeurFlows) is 293,050.

6. A stand-alone table OD _ Neuro _ Flows includes 7,049 records with field NeuroFlows for volumes of neurosurgery patient service flows from each unique residential ZIP code area to each unique neurosurgery hospital ZIP code area. The total volume (i.e., the sum of NeuroFlows) is 40,002.

A separate GIS geodatabase FL _ Ntwk.gdb contains a road network feature dataset FLRd2012, which includes a single feature class also named FLRd2012 for all levels of roads.

Note that the point feature ZIP _ Points is population-weighted centroids of ZIP code areas calibrated from population data at the census block level (Wang, 2015, p.78). The data tables OD _ All _ Flows, OD _ CardNeur _ Flows, and OD _ Neuro _ Flows contain (1) the origin field PatientZipZoneID, identical to the field ZoneID in ZIP _ Code _ Area and ZIP _ points, and (2) the destination field Hosp _ ZoneID, identical to the field Hosp _ ZoneID in Hosp _ ZIP and SPHosp _ ZIP.

Other program files will be discussed when they are first introduced. Other datasets based on other study areas for illustrating some specific tasks will also be explained wherever they are used.

Figure 1.1 shows the study area with population density across ZIP code areas, superimposed with hospitals. Most hospitals are concentrated in metropolitan areas of higher population density.

Refer to the "List of Major Datasets and Program Files" (preceding Chapter 1) for a complete list. The dataset and related programs are needed for the case studies and are accessible via http://faculty.lsu.edu/fahui/.

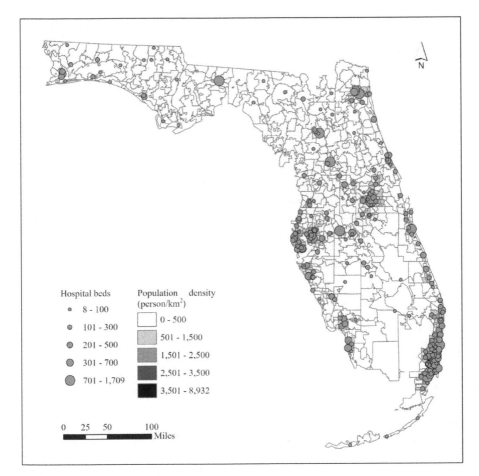

FIGURE 1.1
Spatial distribution of hospitals and ZIP code areas in Florida.

1.4 Overview of Remaining Chapters

Chapters 2 and 3 cover two challenging tasks involved in most of the HSA delineation methods, namely estimating a travel time matrix and deriving the best-fitting distance decay function, respectively. Chapters 4, 5, and 6 introduce three methods for delineating HSAs, namely the refined Dartmouth method, the Huff model, and the network community detection methods, respectively. Chapter 7 discusses the application of delineation of service areas for a specialized health care, cancer care. The following offers a brief overview of these chapters.

Estimating an OD travel time (or distance) matrix is a common task in spatial analysis and is nearly ubiquitous in data preparation in defining functional regions. Chapter 2 introduces various methods for estimating distance and travel time matrices by driving or public transit, in ArcGIS Pro or Google Maps API. When such a matrix is very large, it becomes a major computational challenge. A case study is illustrated to implement the calibration of a nationwide drive time matrix between ZIP code areas in the USA. As trip lengths increase, the volume of OD pairs increases exponentially and our desirable accuracy for estimated drive time declines; therefore, a differential sampling approach is designed to use less-detailed road networks, sample smaller percentages of OD pairs for validation and adjustment, and design algorithms consuming less computational power without much compromising the quality of results. All related algorithms are automated in customized tools and provided for readers to download and practice.

Chapter 3 discusses the distance decay behavior, often referred to as the "first law of geography", in patients seeking medical services. Such a behavior can be captured by various functions on how the volume of patient trips declines with increasing distance or travel time. Obviously, the measure of distance or travel time utilizes results from Chapter 2. This chapter illustrates what functions to consider and how to identify the best-fitting one and examines what we can learn from the variability of the function across subpopulations and across geographic areas. Many spatial analysis tasks, including the Huff model in Chapter 5, rely on the result of derived distance decay function in modeling interactions between the supply and demand sides of a health care market.

Chapter 4 refines the procedure of the Dartmouth method, which pioneered the delineation of HSAs and HRRs in the USA, and introduces a tool that automates the process in ArcGIS Pro. The Dartmouth method uses a simple plurality rule by assigning an area (e.g., a ZIP code area) to a hospital if its residents visit the hospital most often out of alternatives and then collects the areas assigned to the same hospital to form a preliminary HSA. Preliminary HSAs are then adjusted, often manually, to account for spatial adjacency and threshold *localization index (LI)* rate. LI is defined as the fraction of services provided by hospitals within an HSA out of the total service volume generated by patients in the same HSA. Our refined Dartmouth method eliminates the uncertainty and arbitrariness that require interactive decisions by an analyst. The automation not only makes the process efficient, but also ensures that the results are consistent and replicable, two important properties in scientific research. A case study illustrates how to replicate the delineation of Dartmouth HSAs and HRRs in Florida by the automated tool and based on more recent data of all hospitalizations.

Chapter 5 introduces the Huff model and its application in delineating HSAs. The Huff model is best known for deriving trade areas for retail stores, and here it is selected to define HSAs when an analyst only has access to limited data. Data such as the specific patient-to-hospital OD service volumes at a fine geographic scale are often cost-prohibitive (e.g., the HCUP data used in most of the case studies in the book) or require special permissions and user agreements due to the confidential nature of medical data (e.g., the Medicare data used by the Dartmouth Atlas of Health Care Project). The Huff model only needs data such as the locations and sizes of hospitals and residents (or patients) and the transportation networks linking them. It basically estimates the OD service volumes by a gravity-based model and then uses the plurality rule like the Dartmouth method to construct HSAs. The classic Huff model needs to be refined to capture a more realistic spatial behavior of patients and to ensure the spatial contiguity of derived HSAs. A convenient tool is developed in ArcGIS Pro to automate the process. A case study applies the refined Huff model to defining HSAs in Florida and assesses its potential as a proxy method in the absence of OD patient flow data.

Chapter 6 introduces the network community detection approach to delineation of HSAs. A patient-to-hospital OD flow matrix can be treated as a complex network, and the derivation of HSAs becomes a task of segmenting the network into subnetworks (communities). The resulting subnetworks have the maximum connections within each and the minimum connections between them, commonly referred to as "community detection" in network science. Adapting a community detection method for defining HSAs needs to account for some spatial constraints such as area adjacency and threshold population size. This chapter instigates two recently developed methods, based on two popular community detection methods, namely "spatially constrained Louvain and Leiden algorithms". Both are customized in tools in ArcGIS Pro. A case study illustrates and compares the two methods in defining HSAs in Florida to facilitate comparison to those defined by the Dartmouth method.

Chapter 7 applies some of the techniques introduced in other chapters, such as the estimation of a large travel time matrix in Chapter 2, the distance decay effect in Chapter 3, and the network community detection approach in Chapter 6, in delineating the service areas of a specialized health care, cancer care. It also discusses a method of interpolating suppressed OD flow data by a gravity model, a common challenge for similar tasks involving medical data of small numbers. All are illustrated in a case study in the nine-state Northeast Region of the USA.

Among the three methods for HSA delineation, the Dartmouth method or the Huff model usually yields one set of configurated HSAs, unless one changes the constraints or parameters in the method. The network community detection approach delineates a given number of HSAs corresponding to a resolution value defined by the analyst, and the number of derived HSAs rises as the resolution value increases. In other words, the approach is scale-flexible, an important desirable property in regionalization. Perhaps, an analogy can be used to help explain the complex concepts of "community detection" and "scale-flexibility". A network is like a pot of spaghetti full of interconnected strings. Our task is to divide the spaghetti from one pot into a number of bowls gradually. We start with separating it into two bowls by cutting the fewest strings of spaghetti (and thus preserving the maximum number of strings within each bowl). We then continue with the same goal of cutting the fewest strings to divide one of the bowls to two in order to get three bowls of spaghetti. The process continues until we reach the number of bowls (or a certain amount of spaghetti in a bowl) defined by a user. Both network community detection methods show great promises in our pursuit of efficient automation of delineating robust, data-driven, and organic HSAs and represent the state-of-the-art HSA delineation methodology.

In summary, a toolkit with multiple tools is released for delineating HSAs: the Dartmouth method, the Huff model, the two network community detection methods, and several data processing tools that support these HSA delineation methods. The Huff model only requires the data inputs of two layers (facilities and customers) and an optional external distance (or travel time) table between them. The Dartmouth method and the network community detection methods require an additional dataset, namely an OD flow table listing the patient-to-hospital service volumes between the two. Detailed step-by-step implementations of the tools are discussed in the corresponding chapters.

2

Estimating Distance and Travel Time Matrices in GIS

This chapter discusses a fundamental task in spatial analysis: estimating distance and travel time. Defining hospital service areas (HSAs) often requires a distance (or travel time) matrix between patient (resident) locations and hospitals. When a study area is large with a fine spatial resolution, the matrix is large and the task of estimating such a matrix can be challenging.

The very theoretical foundation for forming HSAs is that our travel behavior conforms to the *distance decay rule*, often referred to as the *first law of geography* (Tobler, 1970). Chapter 3 will examine this in detail. One important result from Chapter 3 is the best-fitting distance decay function that captures such a behavior. The function will be fed into the Huff model, discussed in Chapter 5, to delineate HSAs.

This chapter begins with an overview of various measures of spatial impedance from basic distance measures to network travel time in Section 2.1. Section 2.2 focuses on the GIS implementations of calibrating distance and drive time matrices in ArcGIS Pro. Section 2.3 illustrates the process on how to estimate a travel time matrix by transit in ArcGIS Pro. Section 2.4 discusses the use of the Google Maps API to estimate both drive time and transit time matrices. Section 2.5 reports a recent study that integrates some of these skills in estimating a large drive time matrix between ZIP code areas in the USA. The chapter concludes with a brief summary in Section 2.6.

2.1 Measures of Distance and Travel Time

Distance measures include Euclidean distance, geodesic distance, Manhattan distance, network distance, topological distance, and others.

Euclidean distance is simply the distance between two points connected by a straight line on a flat surface. If a study area is small such as a city or a county, Euclidean distance between two points (x_1, y_1) and (x_2, y_2) in Cartesian coordinates is approximated as

$$d_{12} = \left[(x_1 - x_2)^2 + (y_1 - y_2)^2 \right]^{1/2} \tag{2.1}$$

DOI: 10.1201/9780429260285-2

Note that the coordinates are in projected units on a planar surface such as meter or foot, not geographic coordinates such as decimal degrees.

If the study area covers a large territory (e.g., a state or a nation), the geodesic distance is a more accurate measure between two points on the surface of the earth. *Geodesic distance* is the shortest distance between two points through a great circle assuming the earth as a sphere. Given the geographic coordinates of two points as (a, b) and (c, d) in radians, the geodesic distance between them is

$$d_{12} = r * \arccos\left[\sin b * \sin d + \cos b * \cos d * \cos(c - a)\right] \qquad (2.2)$$

where r is the radius of the earth (approximately 6,367.4 km). If the coordinates are in decimal degrees (dd), they need to be converted to radians (rad) as

$$rad = \pi * dd / 180.$$

As the name suggests, *Manhattan distance* describes a rather restrictive movement in rectangular blocks as in the New York City borough of Manhattan. Manhattan distance is the length of the change in the x-direction plus the change in the y-direction. For instance, the Manhattan distance between two nodes (x_1, y_1) and (x_2, y_2) in Cartesian coordinates is computed as

$$d_{12} = |x_1 - x_2| + |y_1 - y_2| \qquad (2.3)$$

Like Euclidean distance, Manhattan distance is only meaningful in a small study area such as a city or county. Manhattan distance is often used as an approximation for network distance if the street network is close to a grid pattern. It has become obsolete in the era of GIS with wide availability of street (road) network data.

Network distance or *network travel time* is the shortest-path distance or travel time through a transportation network. A transportation network consists of a set of nodes (or vertices) and a set of arcs (or edges or links) that connect the nodes, and is usually a directed network as some of the arcs are one-way streets and most of the arcs have two permissible directions. Finding the shortest path from a specified origin to a specified destination is the *shortest-route problem*, which records the shortest distance or the least travel time depending on whether the impedance value is defined as distance or time on each arc. Most algorithms for solving the problem are built upon the popular *label setting algorithm* developed by Dijkstra (1959).

A transportation network has many network elements such as link impedances, turn impedances, one-way streets, overpasses, and underpasses that need to be defined. Putting together a road network requires extensive data collection and processing, which can be very expensive or infeasible for many applications. Section 2.4 discusses some technical details on how to implement it in GIS or use a different approach such as an online routing app (e.g., Google Maps API) to bypass the data preparation.

All the above measures of distance are metric. In contrast, *topological distance* emphasizes the number of connections (edges) between objects instead of their total lengths. For example, the topological distance between two locations on a transportation network is the fewest number of edges that takes to connect them. For the topological distance between polygons, it is 1 between two neighboring polygons, 2 if they are connected through a common neighbor, and so on. Topological distance is used in various centrality indices that measure location advantage in a city (Hillier, 1996) or importance of an entity in a social network (Freeman, 1979). Spatial interaction may also conform to the distance decay rule when distance is measured in topological distance. For example, as reported in Liu et al. (2014), relatedness between provincial units in China declines with increasing topological distances between them.

In a topological network, the edge length between two nodes is coded as 1 if they are directly connected, and 0 otherwise. Topological distances between polygons can be computed by constructing a topological network representing the polygon connectivity, where two adjacent polygons are connected with an edge length of 1. The same shortest-route algorithm for regular distance measure can be used for calibrating topological distances.

Other distance terms such as behavioral distance, psychological distance (e.g., Liberman et al., 2007), mental distance, and social distance emphasize that the aforementioned physical distance measures may not be the best approach to model spatial behavior that varies by individual attributes, by environmental perceptions, and by the interaction between them. For example, one may choose the safest but not necessarily the shortest route to return home, and the choice may be different at various times of the day and vary by individuals. The routes from the same origin to the same destination may differ between a long-term resident with local knowledge and a new visitor to the area.

2.2 Computing Distance and Drive Time Matrices in ArcGIS Pro[1]

Estimating a distance (or travel time) matrix between locations is a critical task in spatial analysis, commonly encountered by researchers in geography, urban planning, transportation engineering, business management, operational research, etc. In this book, the results are fed into analysis of distance

---

[1] For ArcMap users, refer to Wang (2015, p.33–40).

decay behaviors in Chapter 3 and delineation of HSAs by the Huff model in Chapter 5. This section illustrates how the task is implemented step by step in GIS and includes how to estimate a Euclidean or geodesic distance matrix and a drive time matrix.

2.2.1 Computing Euclidean and Geodesic Distance Matrices in ArcGIS Pro

Computing a Euclidean distance matrix or a geodesic distance matrix between any two points either within one layer or between different layers is a common task in ArcGIS. As stated in Section 2.1, one may use Euclidean distance for simplicity in a small study area such as a city or a county, but needs to use geodesic distance to account for the curvature of the earth for better accuracy if the study area is large (e.g., a state or a multi-state region in the USA, or a country).

In ArcGIS Pro, under Analysis, use the tool "Generate Near Table". Define the Input Features and Near Features, and name the Output Table. If it is desirable to have a complete OD matrix from all origins to all destinations, leave the parameter for Search Radius blank and make sure that the option "Find only closest feature" is unchecked and the value for "Maximum number of closest matches" is blank. For the Method, select Planar or Geodesic to calculate Euclidean or geodesic distances, respectively. If one needs the distances between any two points on one feature layer, use that layer to define both the Input Features and the Near Features; the output table has $n*(n-1)$ records, where n represents the number of features in the layer.[2] For a polygon feature, the distances are to the boundary of a polygon feature, not to the centers or centroids of the polygons.

The resulting table includes (1) IN _ FID for the input feature's OBJECTID, (2) NEAR _ FID for the near feature's OBJECTID, (3) NEAR _ DIST for the distance between them, and (4) NEAR _ RANK for the rank of a destination from the nearest to the farthest. Users can join it back to the input feature by the field IN _ FID or the near feature by the field NEAR _ FID. Note that the value of the field NEAR _ DIST has a linear unit of the input feature's coordinate system.[3]

The current ArcGIS Pro version does not have a built-in tool for computing the less commonly used Manhattan distances. Their computation is straightforward by utilizing Equation 2.3 based on projected coordinates in a planar system.

---

[2] The distance matrix does not include the records from any point to itself, and thus n records fewer than $n*n$.

[3] If the input features use a geographic coordinate system, choose Geodesic for Method, and the unit of NEAR _ DIST is meters for the calculated geodesic distance. If one wishes to use the Planar option for the Method parameter to calculate Euclidean distances, the input features need to be projected by using a projection suitable for distance measurement, such as an equidistant projection.

2.2.2 Computing a Drive Time Matrix in ArcGIS Pro

Computing a network distance or travel time matrix by driving utilizes the Network Analysis module in ArcGIS. The task is commonly referred to as "OD Cost Matrix" where the cost (impedance) is defined as length or time of each edge on a network. In other words, cumulating lengths along a route for an OD pair yields its network distance and cumulating time along the route yields its travel time.

(1) Viewing and Preparing the Road Network Source Dataset.

The source feature dataset must have fields representing network impedance values such as distance and travel time. Our network dataset[4] is the feature dataset FLRd2012, currently with only one feature class also named FLRd2012.

In ArcGIS Pro, add the feature dataset[5] FLRd2012 to the project and view its feature class also named FLRd2012 in a map. It contains all levels of roads in Florida. Open its attribute table, and note three fields SPEED, TravelTime, and Shape _ Length. The unit for SPEED is miles per hour (suggested by its values), and the field Shape _ Length is automatically generated by the system with the unit in meters. We can verify that the unit for TravelTime is minutes as "TravelTime = 60 *(!Shape _ Length!/1609)/!SPEED!" when the Expression Type is "Python 3".

(2) Creating and Building the Network Dataset.

On the Analysis tab, in the Geoprocessing pane, click Tools to open the Geoprocessing pane and search for "Create Network Dataset" to locate it. Click on the tool to activate the dialog window. Under Parameters, (1) choose FLRd2012 for Target Feature Dataset, (2) give the name FLRd _ ND for Network Dataset Name, (3) check FLRD2012 for Source Feature Classes, (4) leave the default setting "Elevation fields" for Elevation Model, and (5) click Run to execute the tool. Now under the feature dataset FLRD2012, the newly created network dataset FLRd _ ND and junction feature class FLRd _ ND _ Junctions are added.

Remove the network dataset layer FLRd _ ND from the map so that it can be edited.

In the Catalog pane, right-click the network dataset FLRd _ ND > Properties to open the dialog box, as shown in Figure 2.1. Click Travel Attributes > Costs tab > For Distance; under Properties, you can change the attribute name to Dist _ km and assign Units (Kilometers). Still under Costs tab, click the Menu button ☰ and choose New, and define a new cost field for Time by updating the name to Time _ min and assigning Units (Minutes). Moreover,

---

[4] The network source dataset needs to be a feature dataset so that the other feature classes and data created in the next step can be saved there. If the initial source is a road network as a feature class (or in other formats), create a new feature dataset and import that feature to the dataset.

[5] Do not add the feature dataset to the map directly. One cannot edit any attribute table such as adding a field on an open map.

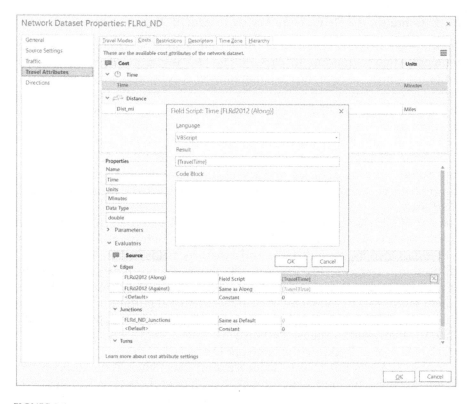

FIGURE 2.1
Network dataset dialog window for travel time setting.

under Evaluators, for FLRd2012 (Along), choose "Field Script" for Type and type "[TravelTime]" in the Field Script dialog window for Result (Figure 2.1). All others are left as default.[6] Click OK to commit the changes.

Now we are ready to build the network. Similarly, in the Geoprocessing pane, search for "Build Network" to locate the tool. Click it to activate the dialog window. Under Parameters, choose the network dataset FLRd _ ND for Input Network Dataset and click Run to execute it. It takes some time to complete the process.[7]

(3) Creating the OD Cost Matrix.

Create a new project. Add the supply and demand feature classes Hosp _ ZIP and ZIP _ Points, and also the newly built network dataset FLRd _ ND to the map. On the Analysis tab, click Network Analysis drop-down menu; under Network Data Source, make sure that the network data source

---

[6] The definitions such as turn, one-way restriction, elevation, accessible intersection, and so on, are left as default for simplicity; the derived travel distance or time matrix is sufficiently accurate for planning purposes.

[7] On a desktop PC of Inter(R) Core(TM) i5-8500 CPU@ 3.00GHz with 16.0GB of memory, it took 7 minutes and 4 seconds to complete the process.

is FLRd _ ND. Click Network Analysis drop-down menu again, and select Origin-Destination Cost Matrix. The OD Cost Matrix layer with several sublayers is added to the Contents pane.

In the Contents pane, click the layer OD Cost Matrix to select it. The OD Cost Matrix tab appears in the Network Analysis group at the top. Click the OD Cost Matrix tab to see the controls including Import Origins, Import Destinations, Travel Settings, and Run, to be defined as below:

a. Click Import Origins to activate the "Add Locations" dialog window. Under Parameters, OD Cost Matrix is Input Network Analysis Layer, Origins is Sub Layer, select ZIP _ Points for Input Locations, input 10000 for Search Tolerance and select Meters as its units.[8] Leave other parameters as default settings. Do not select Append to Existing Locations to avoid generating duplicated records when running this tool for multiple times. Click Run to load the 983 ZIP points as origins.

b. Similarly, click Import Destinations to activate a new "Add Locations" dialog window. Under Parameters, OD Cost Matrix is Input Network Analysis Layer, Destinations is Sub Layer, select Hosp _ ZIP for Input Locations, and use the default 5,000 m for Search Tolerance. Leave other parameters as default settings. Uncheck Append to Existing Locations when running this tool for multiple times. Click Run to load the 213 hospitals as destinations.

c. Open the Travel Settings dialog window. For Travel Mode, name the setting (e.g., auto drive time), choose Driving for Type, define items under Costs (e.g., Time _ min for Impedance, Time _ min for Time Cost, and Dist _ km for Distance Cost), and take the default settings for others. Click OK to accept the settings.

d. Click Run (the first control at the very left) to execute the tool.[9]

In the Contents pane, under the OD Cost Matrix group layer, right-click the sublayer Lines, select Attribute Table to view the result. It contains OriginID and DestinationID that are identical to the field OBJECTID in ZIP _ Points and the field OBJECTID in Hosp _ ZIP, respectively. Export Table to save the result as a table OD _ Time. The number of records is 209,379 (= 983×213).

(4) Saving the OD Drive Time Table.

As stated in Section 1.3, the provided dataset OD _ All _ Flows already includes a field Total _ Time _ min for drive time for the OD pairs between 983 ZIP code areas of patient residences and 213 hospitals. The

---

[8] When using the default Search Tolerance of 5000 m, we would leave out 4 ZIP code points in the coastal south as they are beyond 5 km from their nearest nodes on the road network.
[9] Before executing the tool, make sure that the numbers of origins and destinations match the desirable ones. Do not add either origins or destinations for multiple times, which would add duplicated records to the analysis. On a desktop PC as defined in Footnote 7, the running time is 20 minutes and 14 seconds.

following illustrates how it is derived, which will help the readers practice the technique.

Under Analysis, click Tools to open the Geoprocessing pane, search the tool "Join Field" and use it to (1) append the field ZoneID in ZIP _ Points (common field OBJECTID) to OD _ Time (common field OriginID), and similarly (2) append the field Hosp _ ZoneID in Hosp _ ZIP (common field OBJECTID) to OD _ Time (common field DestinationID). Add a concatenate field Con _ ZoneIDs in Text data type to the table OD _ Time, calculate it by combining ZoneID and Hosp _ ZoneID to define a unique identifier for each OD pair (refer to Figure 2.2).

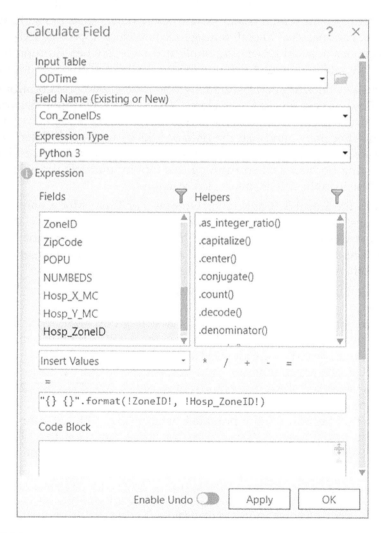

FIGURE 2.2
Dialog window for creating a concatenate field as a unique identifier.

Similarly, add a concatenate field Con _ ZoneIDs to the table OD _ All _ Flows by combining ZoneID and Hosp _ ZoneID to create a unique identifier for each OD pair.

Use "Join Field" again to append the field Total _ Time _ min in the table OD _ Time to OD _ All _ Flows based on the common concatenate field Con _ ZoneIDs in both tables.

2.3 Estimating a Transit Travel Time Matrix in ArcGIS Pro[10]

This section introduces the method for estimating a transit travel time matrix in GIS. Computing a transit travel time matrix is a special scenario of network analysis, which requires a specifically designed transit network dataset. This study uses the *General Transit Feed Specification (GTFS) data model* to describe the fixed-route transit system and then implements the GTFS into the Network Analysis module of ArcGIS Pro to calibrate the OD transit time matrix.

Miami-Dade County in the southeastern Florida is selected as the study area to illustrate the implementation process. Miami-Dade County is one of the largest counties in Florida, with an estimated population of 2.79 million in 2021. Its public transit system is operated by both the City of Miami and Miami-Dade County, with a monthly ridership of more than 7 million (Miami-Dade County Transportation and Public Works, 2019). Excluding the Special Transportation Services (STS), our study covers the other three modes of the Miami-Dade transit system: (1) Metrobus with 95 routes, 9,244 stations, and 2,199 route miles; (2) Metrorail with 2 routes, 23 stations, and 24.8 route miles; and (3) Metromover with 3 routes, 21 stations, and 4.4 route miles (Miami-Dade Transportation Planning Organization, 2018).

The GTFS data for the study area are obtained from the Florida Transit Information System (FTIS) (https://ftis.org/Posts.aspx), saved under the data folder FL _ MDT _ PublicTransit. Also under the folder Florida, the geodatabase FL _ HSA.gdb for this study area has three feature classes ZIP _ Points _ MD, ZIP _ Code _ Area _ MD, and Hosp _ ZIP _ MD representing 80 population-weighted ZIP code points, the associated ZIP code areas, and 21 hospitals, respectively (Figure 2.3).

GTFS is a standardized data format developed by Google to describe fixed-route transit services (Antrim and Barbeau, 2013). It includes a series of tables in the form of comma-delimited text files. These tables use data with pre-defined field names to describe multiple components of a transit system, such as agency information, transit stops and routes, schedules, etc.

[10] Technical help from Dr. Xuan Kuai is gratefully acknowledged in preparing this section.

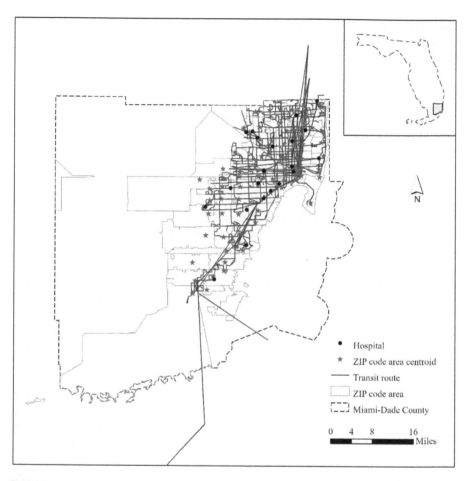

FIGURE 2.3
ZIP code areas, hospitals, and transit routes in Miami-Dade County.

Among those tables, six are necessary to create a functioning GTFS dataset (https://developers.google.com/transit/gtfs/reference):

1. Table `agency.txt` contains basic information about the transit agency, such as its unique ID, full name, URL, and time zone.

2. Table `stops.txt` contains information about each transit stop, such as its ID, name, and geographic coordinates in latitude and longitude.

3. Table `routes.txt` contains information about each transit route, such as its ID, affiliated transit agency ID, short and full names, and type (e.g., bus, subway, ferry).

4. Table `trips.txt` contains information about each transit trip that belongs to every transit route of every transit agency within the transit system, such as its route ID, service calendar ID, and trip ID.

5. Table `stop _ times.txt` contains information about the stop times a vehicle arrives at and departs from each individual transit stop for each individual trip.

6. Table `calendar.txt` or `calendar _ dates.txt` or both. The table `calendar.txt` contains operation calendar types of weekly schedules (e.g., business day only, weekend only, etc.) to be referenced by the transit trips table, while the table `calendar _ dates.txt` contains a set of dates to indicate whether the service is available or not. In general, the two tables are recommended to be used together when some special events, holidays, or school schedules occur on a given date (https://developers.google.com/transit/gtfs/reference#calendartxt).

The following example walks through the entire process of estimating the transit travel time matrix from ZIP code areas to hospitals using the GTFS data of Miami-Dade County in ArcGIS Pro.[11]

(1) Viewing and Preparing the Transit and Road Network Datasets.

Open the data folder `FL _ MDT _ PublicTransit`; there are eight files including the aforementioned six required tables. Open `stop _ times.txt`, and examine the two fields `arrival _ time` and `departure _ time` to ensure no blank values for either. Open `calendar.txt`, examine the two fields `start _ date` and `end _ date` for date ranges and ensure no overlapping, and examine the weekday fields Monday through Sunday with values 1 or 0. Close all txt files.

The street data used here remain the geodatabase `FL _ Ntwk.gdb` containing a road network feature dataset `FLRd2012`, which includes a single feature class also named `FLRd2012`. It is the same road network dataset used in the previous Sub-section 2.2.2 for estimating the drive time matrix for the entire state. Add a new project, add the feature class `FLRd2012` to the Map pane, and open the attribute table of `FLRd2012` to review two required fields `RestrictPedestrians` and `ROAD _ CLASS`.[12]

(2) Creating Transit Stops, Lines, and Schedules from the GTFS Data.

In Catalog, right-click `FL _ Ntwk.gdb` > New > Feature Dataset. Name the new feature dataset `FL _ Transit _ FLRd2012`, import the spatial reference of feature dataset `FLRd2012` to define its coordinate system, and click Run to create it.

Under Analysis, click Tools to open Geoprocessing pane, search "GTFS To Network Dataset Transit Sources" and click on it to activate the dialog window. Select `FL _ MDT _ PublicTransit` for the Input GTFS Folders,

---

[11] ArcMap users refer to `AddGTFStoND _ UsersGuide.html` under the data folder `Florida`.
[12] We added the two fields for estimating transit time. Based on the corresponding FCC codes, the field `RestrictPedestrians` is assigned a value 'N' to prohibit pedestrians for highway and other roads passable only by vehicle, and 'Y' otherwise. Field `ROAD _ CLASS` indicates road types and is used to configure the walking directions.

FL _ Transit _ FLRd2012 for the Target Feature Dataset, and leave other parameters unchecked. Click Run.

Open the two newly generated feature classes Stops and LineVariantElements in the Map pane. The Stops represent the spatial locations of the transit stops, located on the transit line segments LineVariantElements. Note that LineVariantElements is designed to capture the logical connections of the transit system rather than the actual geographic paths driven by buses, trains, or other public transit vehicles.

(3) Connecting the Transit Stops to the Streets.

Right-click feature dataset FL _ Transit _ FLRd2012 in the Catalog. Click Import>Feature Class. Select FLRd2012 for the Input Features, and name the Output Feature Class as Streets. Click Run.

Under Analysis, click Tools to open Geoprocessing pane, search "Connect Network Dataset Transit Sources To Streets" and click on it to activate the dialog window. Select FL _ Transit _ FLRd2012 for the Target Feature Dataset, Streets for the Input Streets Features, and 1,000 m for the Search Distance. Click New expression to construct the expression, choose the field RestrictPedestrians, and set the where clause to "is not equal to" and the value to "Y". Click Run.

Add the two newly generated feature classes StopsOnStreets and StopConnectors to the Map pane. Open the attribute table of StopConnectors, and verify that all values of Shape _ Length are non-zero. Zoom in to any transit stop, and see a short straight-line segment represented by the feature StopConnectors connecting the feature Stops to the feature Streets where the intersection is the feature StopsOnStreets.

(4) Creating and Building the Transit Network Dataset

Under Analysis, click Tools to open Geoprocessing pane, search "Create Network Dataset From Template" and click on it to activate the dialog window. Select the provided XML file TransitNetworkTemplate.xml for Network Dataset Template and feature dataset FL _ Transit _ FLRd2012 for Output Feature Dataset. Click Run. It creates a new network dataset TransitNetwork _ ND. Remove it from the Contents pane so that it can be edited.

In the Catalog pane, right-click network dataset TransitNetwork _ ND>Properties to open the dialog window. Click Source Settings>Group Connectivity tab. The Edges contains feature classes LineVariantElements, StopConnectors, and Streets. The Junctions contains Stops and StopsOnStreets. Under Policy, make sure all three edge sources have Endpoint connectivity, the junction source Stops has the Honor connectivity, and the junction source StopsOnStreets has the Override connectivity. There are three connectivity groups for TransitNetwork _ ND. Under Groups, ensure LineVariantElements in the third groups, StopConnectors in the second groups, and Streets in the first groups. Note that Stops is in the second and third groups to provide a way to transition from connector lines to transit lines, and StopsOnStreets is in the first and second groups to provide a way to transition between the connector lines and streets.

In the Network Dataset Properties dialog window, click Travel Attributes>Costs tab. TransitNetwork _ ND has three cost attributes: PublicTransitTime, WalkTime, and Length. Select PublicTransitTime. Under Evaluators, LineVariantElements (Along) uses Public Transit as Type, and select Constant for the Type of LineVariantElements (Against) and set the Value as -1 to indicate that the traversal is not allowed in the backward direction of the road network. For StopConnectors (Along) and StopConnectors (Against), select Constant for the Type and set the Value as 0.25 to assume that the boarding and exiting time is around 0.25 minutes. For Streets (Along) and Streets (Against), select Field Script for the Type and [Shape_Length]/83.3333 for the Value to assume that 83.3333 m per minute is the default walking speed defined in the Travel Modes tab. Since we are only interested in the PublicTransitTime, keep the default settings for the other two cost attributes.

Under the Travel Attributes, click the Restrictions tab. TransitNetwork _ ND has two restrictions: PedestrianRestriction and WheelchairRestriction. Click PedestrianRestriction; the Usage Type is Prohibited; under Evaluators, Streets (Along) has a Field Script for the Type and the Value defined as !RestrictPedestrians!=="Y", and the same is for Streets (Against). Click WheelchairRestriction; under Evaluators, StopConnectors has a Field Script, and leave the default value for Prohibited.

Under the Travel Attributes, click the Travel Modes tab. There are two available travel modes, "Public transit time" and "Public transit time with wheelchair".[13] Here we only use the first one. Select "Public transit time", ensure that "PublicTransitTime" is the Impedance under the Costs section, it has false values for the last two parameters, "Traveling with a bicycle" and "Traveling with a wheelchair" under the Cost Parameters section, and only PedestrianRestriction is checked under the Restrictions section. Leave default values for other parameters. Click OK to close the Network Dataset Properties dialog window.

Now we are ready to build the transit network. Similarly, in the Geoprocessing pane, search for "Build Network" to locate the tool and click it to activate the dialog window. Under Parameters, choose the network dataset TransitNetwork _ ND for Input Network Dataset and click Run to execute it.

The next step is to implement the network analysis on the newly defined transit network dataset. Its implementation is similar to that with a regular road network as illustrated in Sub-section 2.2.2.

---

[13] More detailed settings of parameters in travel mode, "Public transit time with wheelchair", are available via https://pro.arcgis.com/en/pro-app/latest/help/analysis/networks/create-and-use-a-network-dataset-with-public-transit-data.htm

(5) Creating the OD Cost Matrix.

Create a new project. Add the supply and demand feature classes Hosp _ ZIP _ MD and ZIP _ Points _ MD, and the network dataset TransitNetwork _ ND to the map. On the Analysis tab, click Network Analysis drop-down menu; under Network Data Source, make sure that the network data source is TransitNetwork _ ND. Click Network Analysis drop-down menu again, and select Origin-Destination Cost Matrix. The OD Cost Matrix layer with several sublayers is added to the Contents pane. Click the layer OD Cost Matrix to select it. The OD Cost Matrix tab appears in the Network Analysis group at the top. Define parameters as below:

a. Click Import Origins to activate the "Add Locations" dialog window. Under Parameters, OD Cost Matrix is Input Network Analysis Layer, Origins is Sub Layer, and select ZIP _ Points _ MD for Input Locations. Leave other parameters as default settings. Do not select Append to Existing Locations to avoid generating duplicated records when running this tool for multiple times. Click Run to load the 80 ZIP points as origins.

b. Similarly, click Import Destinations to activate a new "Add Locations" dialog window. Under Parameters, OD Cost Matrix is Input Network Analysis Layer, Destinations is Sub Layer, and select Hosp _ ZIP _ MD for Input Locations. Leave other parameters as default settings. Do not select Append for the same reason. Click Run to load the 21 hospitals as destinations.

c. Open the Travel Settings dialog window. For Travel Mode, name the setting (e.g., public transit time), choose Other for Type, define items under Costs (e.g., PublicTransitTime for Impedance and Time Cost), and take the default settings for others. Click OK to accept the settings.

d. In the Date and Time tab, select Day of Week, 8AM, and Monday, for example.

e. Click Run to execute the tool.[14]

In the Contents pane, under the OD Cost Matrix group layer, right-click the sublayer Lines > Attribute Table to view the result. It contains OriginID and DestinationID that are identical to the field OBJECTID in ZIP _ Points _ MD and the field OBJECTID in Hosp _ ZIP _ MD, respectively. Export the table to save the result as a table OD _ MD _ Pubtransittime.

(6) Preparing Data for Comparing Drive Times and Transit Times.

Here we add an extra step to compare the drive times estimated from Sub-section 2.2.2 and transit times calibrated above. The travel time ratios

---

[14] There are warnings under the Solve message to show that no destinations were found for some origins. Therefore, fewer than $80 \times 21 = 1,680$ OD pairs are retained.

between the two modes play an important role in affecting transit ridership (Kuai and Wang, 2020).

Similar to step 4 in Sub-section 2.2.2, under Analysis, click Tools to open the Geoprocessing pane, search the tool "Join Field" and use it to (1) append the field ZoneID in ZIP _ Points _ MD (common field OBJECTID) to OD _ MD _ Publictransittime (common field OriginID), and similarly (2) append the field Hosp _ ZoneID in Hosp _ ZIP _ MD (common field OBJECTID) to OD _ MD _ Publictransittime (common field DestinationID). Add a concatenate field Con _ ZoneIDs in Text data type to the table OD _ MD _ Publictransittime, and calculate it by combining ZoneID and Hosp _ ZoneID to define a unique identifier for each OD pair. If needed, refer Figure 2.2.

Use "Join Field" again to append the field Total _ Time _ min in OD _ All _ Flows to OD _ MD _ Publictransittime (common field Con _ ZoneIDs in both tables).

The following analysis is based on the two fields Total _ PublicTransitTime for transit time and Total _ Time _ min for drive time in the updated table OD _ MD _ Publictransittime.

Figure 2.4 shows the average transit-to-driving travel time ratios across ZIP code areas in Miami-Dade County, where the values in parentheses represent the numbers of ZIP code areas in corresponding ranges of travel time ratios. Driving a private vehicle is much faster and more convenient across the study area as riding the public transit involves time spent on walking, waiting, boarding and deboarding, and also with a typically slower speed. The disadvantage is even more pronounced with higher travel time ratios in the northwest of Miami-Dade County than elsewhere. In the northeast and south of Miami-Dade County, the travel time ratios are lower as those areas have more bus routes and stops, and the public transit is a more attractive choice for residents in those neighborhoods. Figure 2.5 shows a nonlinear trend that the transit time increases with drive time, but the increasing rate levels off for longer trips. In other words, with comparison to driving, the disadvantage by transit is not as pronounced for longer trips.

2.4 Estimating Drive Time and Transit Time Matrices by Google Maps API

In 2005, Google launched the Google Maps API to allow customization of online maps. The Google Maps API enables one to estimate the travel time without reloading the Web page or displaying portions of the map. An earlier version of a Python program was developed to use the Google Maps API for computing an OD travel time matrix (Wang and Xu, 2011). An improved

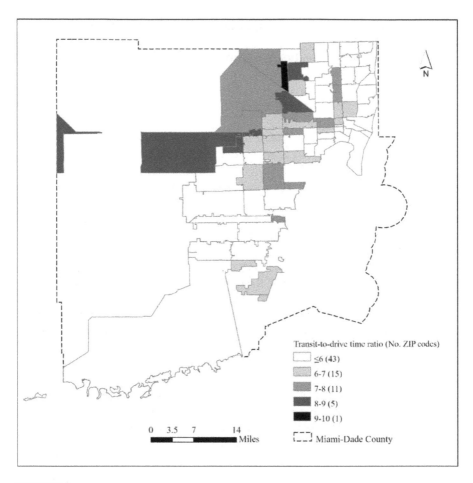

FIGURE 2.4
Transit-to-drive time ratios for ZIP code areas in Miami-Dade County.

version `GoogleODTravelTimePro.py`, available under the subfolder `Scripts`, is used here to illustrate its usage.

The program reads the origin (O) and destination (D) layers of point or polygon features in a projected coordinate system and automatically calculates the latitudes and longitudes of all features by their point locations or geographic centroids of the polygons. The data are fed into a tool in Python that automates the process of estimating the travel time and distance matrix between a set of origins and a set of destinations at a time by calling the Google Maps Distance Matrix API. The iterations stop when the program reaches the last OD combination. The result is saved in an ASCII file (with a file extension .txt) listing each origin, each destination, travel time (in *minutes*), and distance (in *miles*) between them. The origins and destinations are represented by the OBJECTIDs of the input features, which can be used to link the travel time result.

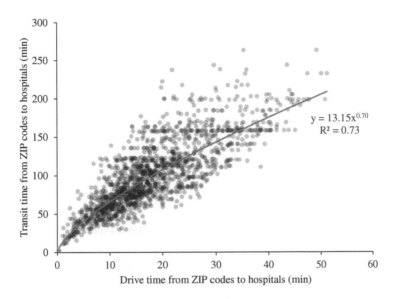

FIGURE 2.5
Drive time vs transit time from ZIP code areas to hospitals in Miami-Dade County.

Before using this service, an API key is needed to authenticate each request associated with this program.[15] We randomly selected 10 ZIP codes and 10 hospitals in Miami-Dade County, Florida, as origins and destinations, and thus 100 OD pairs to demonstrate the tool's use. The program can be added to ArcGIS Pro as a tool, and the following steps illustrate its implementation.

1. Create a new project with the Catalog template. Under the Contents, right-click Toolboxes > Add Toolbox. In the dialog window "Add Toolbox", navigate to the "Florida" folder, select "Google API Pro.tbx", and click OK to add it.

2. Click the newly added Toolbox "Google API Pro.tbx". Under the Catalog pane, right-click the script named "Google OD Travel Time" and select Properties to activate the Tool Properties dialog window. Under General, click Browse ▨ on the right side of the Script File, navigate to the "Scripts" folder, and select GoogleODTravelTimePro.py.

3. Under the Tool Properties > Parameters, define the five parameters (API Key, Input Features as Origins, Input Features as Destinations,

---

[15] Readers must go to the Google Cloud Platform Console to create a project with a billing account to enable the service of Distance Matrix API and then create an API key. The Google Maps Platform uses a pay-as-you-go pricing model. It provides a $200 free monthly credit that allows 40,000–50,000 OD records per month, enough to support this case study. Visit https://developers.google.com/maps/documentation/distance-matrix/overview?hl=zh_CN for more detail.

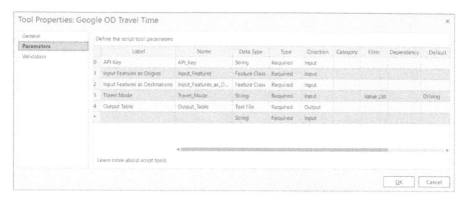

FIGURE 2.6
Dialog window for defining Tool Properties of Google OD Travel Time.

Travel Mode, and Output Table in Data Type of String, Feature Class, Feature Class, String, and Text File, respectively, as shown in Figure 2.6). All parameters are required, and the former four parameters have a Direction of Input and the last one has a Direction of Output. For the Travel Mode, select Value List for Filter. In the Value List Filter dialog window, add Driving and Transit and click OK to close the window. Select Driving for Default, and click OK to close the Tool Properties dialog window.

4. Double-click the script "Google OD Travel Time" under the "Google API Pro.tbx"[16] to activate the program in the Geoprocessing pane.

As shown in Figure 2.7, a user needs to input the Google API key, two point or polygon features in projected coordinate systems as origin and destination, and a text file name as the result. In this case, we select two point feature classes ZIP _ Points _ MD10 and Hosp _ ZIP _ MD10 under the geodatabase FL _ HSA.gdb for the "Input Features as Origins" and "Input Features as Destinations", respectively, which represent 10 randomly selected ZIP codes and 10 randomly selected hospitals in Miami-Dade County. We name the text files as (1) ZIP _ Hosp _ DriveTime.txt when Driving is chosen for the Travel Mode, and (2) ZIP _ Hosp _ TransitTime.txt when Transit is chosen for the Travel Mode. The total computational time depends on the size of OD travel time matrix, the performance of the running computer, the Internet connection speed, and the request limit.[17]

---

[16] You can click "Google API Pro.tbx" to use it directly. If it is desirable to have it loaded by default every time you open ArcGIS Pro, right click "Google API Pro.tbx" and select "Add to Favorites".

[17] See details on the billing via https://developers.google.com/maps/documentation/distance-matrix/usage-and-billing. For the case study, it took us approximately 15 and 21 seconds for the two travel time matrices on a desktop of Intel(R) Xeon(R) Gold 6140 CPU @ 2.30GHz with 128GB RAM.

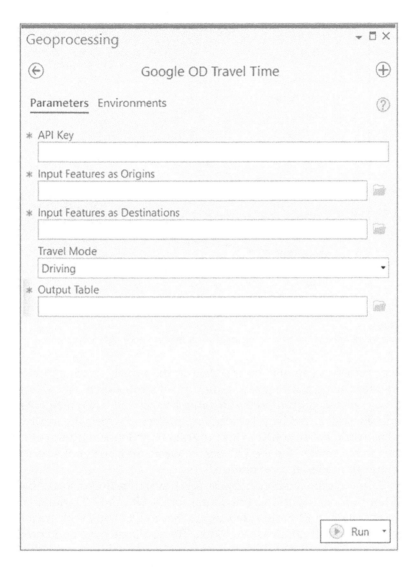

FIGURE 2.7
Google Maps API tool user interface for computing OD travel time matrix.

Note that some OD trips derived from the transit mode may have blank values for travel time and distance. When neither the departure_time nor the arrival_time is specified in the request, the departure_time defaults to the current time running the program, which may happen to have no public transit in operation for the routes. In addition, the Google Maps Distance Matrix API provides multiple transit modes, such as bus, subway, train, rail, and tram, which can be specified in the transit_mode parameter as one or more composite modes of transit. The preferences such as less_walking

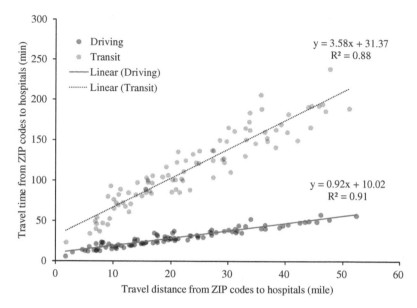

FIGURE 2.8
Travel distance vs. travel time by driving and transit modes via Google Maps.

and fewer_transfers can also be specified in the transit_routing_preference parameter for the transit requests. Other travel modes such as walking and bicycling are also supported in the Distance Matrix API when the pedestrian paths and sidewalks, and bicycle paths and preferred streets are available on the road network. For simplicity, this program only defines driving or transit in the mode parameter for the OD trip requests and does not specify any detailed transit modes and preference.[18]

Figure 2.8 shows the relationship between travel time and distance by driving and transit modes with two fitted lines for the 93 valid OD trips from ZIP codes to hospitals in Miami-Dade County. Seven OD trips with travel time and distance in blank values are excluded. Travel distance is a good predictor for travel time for both travel modes, and understandably it is a better predictor for drive time with $R^2=0.91$ than transit time with $R^2=0.88$. The transit time includes waiting, walking, and transition times that are not necessarily related to distance. The fitted line has a significantly higher intercept (31.37 vs. 10.02) and a much steeper slope (3.58 vs. 0.92) for transit than those for driving. In other words, transit riders need to allocate a much longer fixed time regardless of trip lengths (given less flexible departure time) and even more variable time (about three times more) as trip lengths increase.

It is also valuable to compare the driving and transit times estimated by the Google Maps API to those by ArcGIS Pro in Sub-section 2.2.2 and Section

---

[18] More details about transportation mode in Distance Matrix API can be found via https://developers.google.com/maps/documentation/distance-matrix/overview.

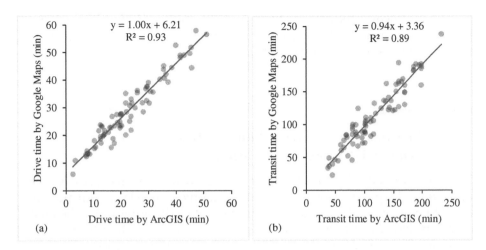

FIGURE 2.9
(a) Drive time and (b) transit time by ArcGIS and Google Maps.

2.3. As shown in Figure 2.9a and b,[19] the estimated drive and transit times by the two are largely consistent with $R^2=0.93$ and 0.89, respectively. Both travel times derived by the Google Maps API are longer than those estimated by ArcGIS, consistent with the findings from Wang and Xu (2011). The driving and transit times have significant intercepts of 6.21 and 3.36 minutes, respectively, which probably reflect the elements of starting and ending times on a trip for getting on to and off the road network, not captured by ArcGIS. For drive time, a slope of 1.0 indicates that Google times can simply be obtained by adding a constant to ArcGIS times. For transit time, a slope of 0.94 indicates that Google times for longer trips regress to better match ArcGIS times, and the adjustment may not be as straightforward. Given the relatively small sample size, we refrain from further generalization.

One may favor the Google Maps API approach as it accounts for the actual traffic condition in both driving and transit modes and thus yields more realistic estimates. It also has advantages such as the convenience of not preparing a road network dataset and the ability of tapping into Google's updated road data and algorithm. It is also desirable to specify an individual's preferences, such as the departure time and (or) arrival time, avoiding the use of ferry, highway, and tolls, and preferring a limited amount of walking or transfers, which is of great help to derive more favorable travel time and distance based on actual needs. However, it also has some major limitations. The most important is Google's request limit, which may not meet the demand of many spatial analysis tasks. The computational time also seems long. Another drawback for many advanced researchers is that a user has

---

[19] There are 78 valid OD trips as some destination hospitals are not found for some origin ZIP code areas.

neither control over the data quality nor any editing rights. Furthermore, the tool can only generate the current travel time and thus is not suitable for work that needs the travel time in the past.

2.5 Estimating a Large Drive Time Matrix by a Differential Sampling Approach

Sections 2.2 and 2.4 illustrate how to calibrate a drive time matrix by ArcGIS and Google Maps API. However, when the matrix is large (e.g., with millions of OD pairs), it can be a time-consuming and challenging task. The challenges include availability of reliable road network (including traffic) data, programming expertise for automation, and computational power. This section uses a case study of estimating a very large drive time matrix between ZIP code areas in the USA to introduce a differential sampling method. The method is reported in a recent paper by Hu et al. (2020). Here it is adapted with an emphasis on explaining the conceptual model.

The method uses algorithms of varying complexity and computational time to estimate drive times of different trip lengths and can be implemented on a desktop computer. It utilizes the skills introduced such as calibration of a geodesic distance matrix in Sub-section 2.2.1 and estimations of a drive time matrix by ArcGIS in Sub-section 2.2.2 and by Google Maps API in Section 2.4, and offers readers another opportunity to develop an in-depth understanding of those techniques. ZIP code area is a popular geographic unit used in many nationwide datasets in the USA, such as the Healthcare Cost and Utilization Project (HCUP) data used in this book. The result of a derived ZIP-to-ZIP drive time matrix can be a useful resource for spatial analysis of health studies in the USA.

In an OD matrix for a study area, as it is the case for the ZIP-to-ZIP matrix in the USA, the number of OD pairs usually increases significantly as the distance range increases and a user's desirability of accuracy for travel time estimation declines as travelers are less sensitive to a minor difference in trip time. The design of our *differential sampling method* is built upon this behavior. As trip lengths increase, the method requires less data preparation and uses less computational power without much compromising the quality of results. As the number of OD pairs goes up rapidly with rising trip lengths, saving in computational time becomes even more significant. To improve the estimation for those long-range trips, we only use a more accurate method (e.g., via the Google Maps API) to estimate a small fraction of their OD trips by random sampling, derive a set of empirical models on the relationship between preliminary lower-computational-cost estimates and the more accurate estimates, and adjust the preliminary estimates accordingly. As trip lengths increase, computational complexity declines and the sampling intensity also drops.

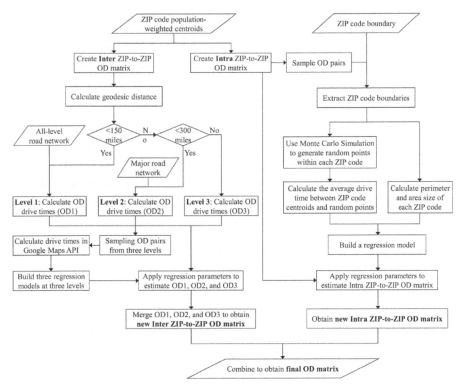

FIGURE 2.10
Conceptual model for estimating a ZIP-to-ZIP drive time matrix in the USA.

Figure 2.10 outlines the workflow for the conceptual model. The process includes three major steps: (1) obtaining a preliminary estimate of the centroid-to-centroid drive times between every two ZIP code areas, which is also named as Inter ZIP-to-ZIP OD matrix, (2) using the Google Maps API to derive drive times for randomly sampled OD pairs and adjusting the Inter ZIP-to-ZIP drive time matrix based on regression models, and (3) incorporating the intra-zonal drive times associated with both origin and destination ZIP code areas, termed "Intra ZIP-to-ZIP OD matrix", to finalize the estimation. Each step is elaborated below.

2.5.1 Estimating Preliminary Inter-zonal Times

Based on geodesic distances, we divide all OD pairs into three levels with different ranges of trip lengths.

1. For *Level 1*, namely short trips with geodesic distance < 150 miles, the OD drive times are computed by ArcGIS by utilizing all levels of roads (including interstates, US and state highways, major roads, and local roads) in routing.

2. For *Level 2*, namely medium-range trips with geodesic distance 150–300 miles, the OD drive times are completed by ArcGIS via major roads (including only interstates, and US and state highways).

3. For *Level 3*, namely long trips with geodesic distance ≥ 300 miles, we simply use the geodesic distances with a constant 50 mph speed to establish a baseline estimate of drive times.

As summarized in Table 2.1, the number of OD pairs increases from Level 1 to 2 and 3, with Level 3 accounting for close to 90% of all OD pairs. The computational time for one OD pair declines from Level 1 to Level 2 as the road network becomes simpler and is negligible for mere geodesic distance computation for Level 3. The accuracy in derived preliminary drive times also declines from Level 1 to 2 and 3.

2.5.2 Calibrating Inter-zonal Times on Randomly Sampled OD Pairs by Google Maps API

This step improves the estimates by using the Google Maps API to account for actual experiences on the road including traffic condition. Due to cost concerns (both financially and timewise), we apply it only to a small subset of randomly sampled OD pairs. As reported in Table 2.1, the sampling ratio declines from Level 1 to 2 and 3. The sampling intensity for Level 1 is about triple those for Level 2 and quadruple those for Level 3. Obviously, better accuracy demands a higher ratio of sampling. Oversampling shorter trips is to enhance their representation and ensure the quality of subsequent interpolation for greater interests by users in acquiring shorter-range travel times. The drop in the sampling ratio is more noticeable from Level 1 to Level 2, but to a less degree from Level 2 to Level 3. Our rationale is that the loss in estimate accuracy is to a less extent from Level 1 to Level 2 as the road network has less detail, in comparison with the change from using network travel times in Levels 1 and 2 to geodesic distances in Level 3. In other words, it is to moderate the loss of accuracy from Level 2 to Level 3 attributable to the decline in sampling

TABLE 2.1

Frequency Distribution of OD Pairs for Levels 1–3

Level	All OD Pairs		Sampling Pairs		Sampling % (n_{sample}/n)
	Count (n)	%	Count (n_{sample})	%	
1	28,241,488	2.62	11,684	9.40	0.041
2	80,547,438	7.47	11,365	9.14	0.014
3	969,643,834	89.91	101,301	81.46	0.010
Total	1,078,432,760	100.00	124,350	100.00	0.012

TABLE 2.2

Regression Models on the Improved Estimates of Drive Time

	Level 1	Level 2	Level 3
Intercept	5.69[a] (16.65)	0.32(0.469)	33.91[a] (42.54)
T_{a1}	0.94[a] (347.689)	0.96[a] (375.45)	0.88[a] (1590.26)
N	11,684	11,365	101,301
R^2	0.91	0.93	0.96

Note: T_{a1} represents preliminary drive time estimates, N denotes the number of observations, and t values are in parentheses.
[a] Statistically significant at the 0.001 level.

intensity as a counterbalance to the drop in accuracy attributable to travel time estimation methods.

Based on the sampled OD pairs of preliminary drive time estimates from Sub-section 2.5.1 and improved estimates by Google Maps API, three regression models, corresponding to the three levels of trip ranges, are obtained in Table 2.2.[20] These three empirically derived regression models are then applied to the remaining OD pairs for adjusting the preliminary estimates of drive times.

2.5.3 Appending Intra-zonal Times

Intra-zonal trips (from a ZIP code area to itself) are usually neglected in travel time estimation via a centroid-to-centroid approach (Bhatta and Larsen, 2011). Such an omission can be significant for short trips, especially for large suburban or rural ZIP code areas. We randomly sample a subset of ZIP code areas (320, about 1% of the ZIP code areas nationwide). In each sampled ZIP code area, the Monte Carlo simulation method (Hu and Wang, 2016) is used to generate a number of random points and the average drive time between these points and the ZIP code area centroid is then computed. As suggested by the literature (Horner and Murray, 2012; Hu and Wang, 2019), intra-zonal drive time is positively related to the perimeter and area of a zone. After testing several regression models, the best-fitting one with $R^2=0.96$ is obtained as follows:

$$t_{ii} = -0.02 + 0.04 ZC_{Pi} + 0.88\sqrt{ZC_{Ai}}$$

where intra-zonal time t_{ii} within ZIP code area i is predicted by two explanatory variables, its perimeter ZC_{Pi} and square root of its area size $\sqrt{ZC_{Ai}}$. The

---

[20] Why does the value of R^2 increase from 0.91 for Level 1 to 0.93 for Level 2 and then to 0.96 for Level 3? When the trip length increases, the predictor becomes coarser, but a larger error in absolute value does not necessarily correspond to a larger difference in relative value. In other words, Google times are more sensitive to the effect of traffic condition in shorter-range trips. It once again justifies the soundness of the conceptual model.

formula is then applied to populate intra-zonal drive times for the remaining ZIP code areas.

Finally, the intra-zonal times at both the origin and destination ZIP code areas are appended to the inter-zonal estimates from Sub-section 2.5.2 for updating the entire OD time matrix.

The study reported in Hu et al. (2020) has 32,840 ZIP code areas with non-zero population in the USA, and their locations are the population-weighted centroids based on the 2010 Census block population data. The result is a massive OD cost matrix of 1,078,465,600 ($= 32,840^2$) records, each of which consists of estimation of drive time and distance for a ZIP code pair. It takes about a total of 76 hours for us to compute and export the national ZIP-to-ZIP time matrix, with the breakdowns of 6 hours for Level 1, 60 hours for Level 2, and 10 hours for Level 3.[21]

Readers are encouraged to visit https://geonavilab.geog.ufl.edu/downloads/ to download related program tools and extract desirable data. The tools include those for generating an OD travel time matrix by ArcGIS from a road network and by Google Maps, calibrating inter-zonal or intra-zonal OD matrix, writing OD pairs with geodesic distance, and extracting the ZIP-to-ZIP OD matrix by states, a list of ZIP codes or other parameters. See a detailed user guide in Appendix A.

Note that the ZIP codes in the case study are ZIP code areas with non-zero population and do not include all ZIP codes. Most of those missing ZIP codes have no associated areas such as post office box ZIP codes and single-site ZIP codes (government, building, or large volume customer). The U.S. Postal Service also updates the ZIP codes periodically. Assuming that the location of a missing ZIP code can be approximated by the average of its three nearest ZIP codes, one may use the following algorithm to interpolate the drive times on corresponding missing OD pairs:

1. For drive time between a missing ZIP code (say, origin) and a known ZIP code (say, destination): Identify the three nearest known ZIP codes from the missing ZIP code, locate the three drive times between each of the three nearby known ZIP codes (origin) and the known ZIP (destination) from the provided matrix, and use their average drive time as the one between the missing ZIP code and the known ZIP code.

2. For drive time between two missing ZIP codes: Identify the three nearest known ZIP codes from the origin ZIP code and also the three nearest known ZIP codes from the destination ZIP code, locate the corresponding nine drive times between each of the three nearby origins and each of the three nearby destinations from the provided OD cost matrix, and use their average drive time as the one between the two missing ZIP codes.

---

[21] On a desktop PC with an Intel Core i7 processer and a 16 GB RAM.

For studies being performed in other geographic scales, such as census tract, or other geographic areas, the derived parameters can also be referenced as a baseline. The proposed research method or framework is also useful for one to imitate in a different country (region) of a similar scale.

2.6 Summary

Measuring spatial impedance is an essential task in spatial analysis. Popular measures include Euclidean distance, geodesic distance, and distances and travel times via various transportation modes. This chapter introduced GIS methods for estimating a distance (or travel time) matrix between a set of locations. ArcGIS Pro provides the Generate Near Table tool to derive a Euclidean (or geodesic) distance matrix, and the OD Cost Matrix tool in the Network Analysis module to calibrate a road network distance (or travel time) matrix via driving. Both are considered routine as the software becomes increasingly user-friendly and the related data are widely available.

Estimating a travel time matrix via transit is more challenging for data availability and technical implementation. While the use of public transit is limited in geographic coverage and ridership, especially in the USA, it is an important transportation mode to be considered in many studies (e.g., disparity in spatial accessibility of health care, mobility, risk in exposure to infectious diseases). Most GIS data of transit systems (e.g., in GTFS format) are publicly accessible and can be converted and integrated into ArcGIS with reasonable effort. After the conversion, ArcGIS Pro also provides the OD Cost Matrix tool in the Network Analysis module to calibrate the transit time matrix while accounting for wait time, boarding/alighting time, and onboard travel time.

This chapter also introduced how to use a Web mapping service, Google Maps API, to compute a drive time or transit time matrix. This frees an analyst of the burden of preparing street network data and accessing advanced GIS or transportation software. Moreover, it accounts for the effect of real-time traffic and yields more realistic estimates. Our automated tool makes the task even more convenient. Most of computation requests for a drive or transit time matrix can be accommodated with the free credit offered by Google.

The case study of estimating the large ZIP-to-ZIP drive time matrix in the USA serves three purposes. It provides a conceptual framework for researchers to design their own approach to tackling a similar challenge with limited resources. It also illustrates how to improve the estimates from three popular methods (calibrating geodesic distances in a simple function, estimating drive time in ArcGIS, and extracting drive time via Google Maps API) by empirically derived regression models. Furthermore, the related program tools and results (e.g., extracting a ZIP-to-ZIP drive time matrix for a specific set of states or region) can be a valuable resource for users.

3

Analysis of Spatial Behavior of Health Care Utilization in Distance Decay

The *distance decay rule* demonstrates that the interaction effect between physical or socioeconomic objects declines with the distance between them. It is also referred to as Waldo R. Tobler's (1970) *first law of geography*, which states that "all things are related, but near things are more related than far things". The distance decay rule captures a fundamental spatial behavior in many aspects of our daily life, such as commuting for work (De Vries et al., 2009), shopping (Young, 2005), or recreation activities (Năstase et al., 2019).

This chapter focuses on such a behavior in utilizing health care services. Examining the behavior in distance decay is important. It reflects a patient's travel burden in access to care, and a longer trip may discourage one's enrollment in the service (Onega et al., 2009a) and lead to negative outcomes (Onega et al., 2009b). However, a wider travel range in seeking medical cares for a demographic group may also reflect their higher mobility and more choices in cares, and thus being more advantageous in competing for quality cares. The result from analysis of such a distance decay behavior serves as the foundation for other spatial analysis tasks. For example, the Huff model in Chapter 5 relies on a distance decay function derived from this chapter to estimate the probability of residents choosing a hospital among others. The distance decay function that best captures patients' spatial behavior is also critical in measuring the spatial accessibility of health care for residents, predicting the impacts of hospital closures or openings on workload for hospital staff, and others.

This chapter has five sections. Section 3.1 overviews various functions in modeling distance decay. Section 3.2 outlines the values of related analysis. Section 3.3 discusses the spatial interaction model approach to deriving the best-fitting distance decay function and a case study of examining the variability of distance decay effect in hospitalization across geographic areas in Florida. Section 3.4 introduces another approach, namely the complementary cumulative distribution curve, to deriving the best function, and uses the same case study to illustrate how the function varies across population groups. Section 3.5 concludes the chapter with a summary.

DOI: 10.1201/9780429260285-3

3.1 Distance Decay Functions

In a review paper on modeling health care accessibility, Wang (2012) summarizes various ways of conceptualizing the distance decay function $f(d)$ in the literature. As illustrated in Figure 3.1, it can be

1. a continuous function such as power (exponential) as in Figure 3.1a or normal as in Figure 3.1b,
2. a discrete set of stepwise values such as 1–0 binary as in Figure 3.1c or multiple stepwise values as in Figure 3.1d, or
3. a hybrid of the two such as a kernel function (i.e., a continuous function within a certain distance range and a fixed value beyond) as in Figure 3.1e or a three-zone hybrid (i.e., a continuous function in the middle and a fixed value within a short range or beyond a long range) as in Figure 3.1f.

This book focuses on continuous functions as an analytical way to capture the full spectrum of variability. Some continuous distance decay functions commonly found in the literature include:

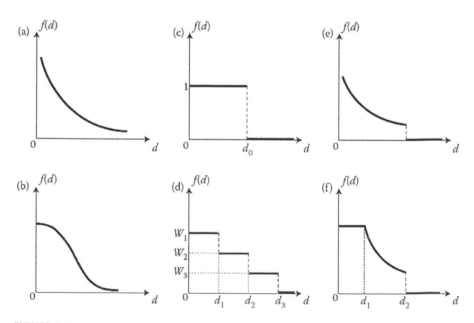

FIGURE 3.1
Conceptualization of distance decay function $f(d)$: (a) power or exponential, (b) normal, (c) binary, (d) multiple stepwise, (e) kernel, and (f) three-zone hybrid.

1. the *power function* $f(d) = d^{-\beta}$ (e.g., Hansen, 1959),
2. the *exponential function* $f(d) = e^{-\beta d}$ (e.g., Wilson, 1969),
3. the *square-root exponential function* $f(d) = e^{-\beta\sqrt{d}}$ (e.g., Taylor, 1983),
4. the *Gaussian function* $f(d) = \frac{1}{\sigma\sqrt{2\pi}} e^{-\frac{1}{2}\left(\frac{d-\mu}{\sigma}\right)^2}$ (e.g., Shi et al., 2012), and

    when $\mu=0$ and simplifying the constant terms, it becomes the *normal function* $f(d) = e^{-\beta d^2}$, and
5. the *log-normal function* $f(d) = e^{-\beta(\ln d)^2}$ (e.g., Taylor, 1983).
    All the above five functions contain one parameter β, often referred to as the *distance friction coefficient*, while others consider more complicated forms, such as:
6. the *log-logistic function* $f(d) = 1/\left(1 + (d/\alpha)^\beta\right)$ (e.g., Delamater et al., 2013), and
7. the *compound power-exponential function* $f(d) = e^{-\alpha d^\beta}$ (Halás et al., 2014).

Both the log-logistic and compound power-exponential functions contain two parameters: α and β, and it is not a fair comparison in fitness of power such as R^2 between these two-parameter functions (6–7) and those simple one-parameter functions (1–5).

As stated in Chapter 2, regardless of the measure of spatial impedance d in distance, travel time, or cost, the effect is simply called "distance decay". There are also many benefits on the theoretical front as well as practical applications to capture the spatial behavior of health care utilization by a distance decay function in place of a simple measure such as average distance or time. A function is an analytical way to model the whole spectrum of health care seekers who exhibit different travel ranges by choice or out of necessity. It is more realistic and informative while maintaining its simplicity. For example, a single distance friction coefficient β in any of the five one-parameter distance decay functions reflects the mobility of travelers.

3.2 Value of Analyzing Distance Decay Effects in Health Care Studies

This section outlines some important roles a distance decay function plays in issues discussed in subsequent chapters of the book and other related works in health care studies.

First, it helps us advance the understanding of classic *central place theory* (Christaller, 1966), the theoretical foundation for a hierarchal system where smaller HSAs are nested within larger HRRs. The classic central place theory partitions a region into a set of hierarchical hexagonal lattices, and each hexagon serves as a market area of a service center at that level. Two critical concepts in the theory are *threshold population,* which is the minimum number of patrons needed for a business in that market area to be sustainable, and *range,* which represents a maximum distance that patrons are willing to travel to acquire its service. A higher order of service (e.g., cardiovascular and neural surgeries by a tertiary hospital that anchors an HRR) requires a larger threshold population in a larger market area than a lower order of service (e.g., regular hospitalization by a general hospital at the center of an HSA). The center of a market area at any level is also the center of the lower-level market area(s) served by that center, which allows centers to provide multiple levels of services and minimizes the total number of centers required in the system. In the context of a hospital system, a tertiary hospital serving a large region also provides other general services to a small region around it, and in addition to that small region, the large region is composed of multiple lower-order service areas served by their respective central general hospitals. Therefore, multiple and smaller HSAs anchored by general hospitals form a larger HRR anchored by more specialized services.

However, the classic central place theory assumes fixed distance ranges for corresponding services, and this rigid confinement cannot account for the diverse spatial behavior of customers choosing the same service. Jia et al. (2017b) argued that a more realistic characterization of spatial behavior for patients seeking different levels of hospital services is their differing travel friction coefficients in a distance decay function. General patients experience a steeper gradient and thus a shorter average travel range, and they form HSAs, whereas specialized patients exhibit a flatter gradient and thus a longer average travel range, and they form HRRs. Therefore, the number of HSAs is larger than that of HRRs, and each HSA has a smaller area size than each HRR. This is a significant advancement from the classic central place theory and solidifies the theoretical foundation for a two-tiered hierarchal health care system of HSAs and HRRs.

Secondly, a distance decay function is a critical element in estimating spatial interaction between residents and health care facilities in the form of patient service flows. In the absence of OD patient flow data, the Huff model in Chapter 5 relies on the locations and sizes of population and hospitals and the distance decay function between them to estimate such data. Even when such data exist, privacy concerns mandate suppression of records of small numbers for protected medical data. For example, Wang et al. (2020) utilized the cancer service flows between ZIP code areas from the Medicare data to analyze the network structure of cancer care market. A major challenge was the suppression of records for service volumes less than 11, which accounted for the majority (about 65%) of total records. With such a significant portion of edges with missing weights, most of which were in short range, the network appeared highly fragmented and any delineation of HSAs without imputation of those suppressed small values would not be meaningful. The strategy used by that study was to estimate a spatial interaction model with the best-fitting distance decay function based on the available data (i.e., records for volumes ≥11), and then use the derived model to interpolate the suppressed records that fell within the range of [1,10]. See Section 7.2 for detail.

Thirdly, a distance decay function derived from empirical data can play an important role in defining the "modularity" of spatial networks in some algorithms for network community detection. *Modularity*, a common quality measure of network partition, is usually formulated as the difference between actual and expected connectivity (e.g., sum of all edge weights) (see Chapter 6 for more detail). A higher modularity value indicates a better partition of network communities. Expert et al. (2011) proposed a modularity function by incorporating the gravity model to capture more realistic expected (or estimated) flows for a spatial network. The purpose of doing so is to improve the measurement of expected connectivity since a spatial network has various spatial constraints (e.g., geography, real-world transport networks, weak or no connections for long-distance links). Gao et al. (2013) adopted a similar strategy, but used the ratio of actual flows over estimated flows in place of absolute value of difference between the two used by Expert et al. (2011). The refinement on the modularity measure by Gao et al. (2013) was to detect small communities, which were more sensitive to the ratio change than large communities. Both studies derived a distance decay function from empirical data to define the gravity model.

There are also ample of issues beyond HSA delineation where a reliable distance decay function needs to be defined in order to capture the spatial behavior of patients in utilizing health care services. Here we use a closely related issue to further highlight its value. A popular method in the literature for measuring spatial accessibility of health care is the *two-step floating catchment area* (*2SFCA*) *method* (Luo and Wang, 2003; Wang, 2012). In step 1, for each supply location, sum up the surrounding demands that are discounted by a distance decay function across all demand locations and compute the supply to summed-up demand ratio there. In step 2, for each demand location, sum up the ratios derived from step 1, discounted by a distance decay function again, across all supply locations, to obtain the accessibility at that demand location. In essence, the method is basically a ratio between supply and demand of a service, which interact with each other via a distance decay effect. Various modifications proposed on the method have centered at different ways of conceptualizing distance decay in patient–physician interactions. Any debate over the best function for distance decay "cannot be settled without analyzing real-world health care utilization behavior" (Wang, 2012, p. 1107). The same applies for its inverted version, *inverted two-step floating catchment area* (*i2SFCA*) *method*, that measures potential crowdedness of facilities (Wang, 2018). See Table 3.1 for a brief recap on both methods. In short, a

TABLE 3.1

Implementing 2SFCA versus i2SFCA

	2SFCA	i2SFCA
Objective	Measuring spatial accessibility of service by residents at demand location i	Measuring potential crowdedness at supply location j
Step 1	For each supply location j, sum up surrounding demands D_k, discounted by distance decay function $f(d_{kj})$, across all demand locations k (=1, 2, ..., m), and compute the supply-to-demand ratio R_j: $R_j = S_j / \sum_{k=1}^{m}\left(D_k f\left(d_{kj}\right)\right)$	For each demand location i, sum up supplies S_l, discounted by distance decay function $f(d_{il})$, across all supply locations l (=1, 2, ..., n), and compute the demand-to-supply ratio r_i: $r_i = D_i / \sum_{l=1}^{n}\left(S_l f\left(d_{il}\right)\right)$
Step 2	For each demand location i, sum up ratios R_j, discounted by distance decay function $f(d_{ij})$, across all supply locations j (=1, 2, ..., n), to yield accessibility A_i at demand location i: $A_i = \sum_{j=1}^{n}\left[R_j f\left(d_{ij}\right)\right]$ $= \sum_{j=1}^{n}\left[S_j f\left(d_{ij}\right) / \sum_{k=1}^{m}\left(D_k f\left(d_{kj}\right)\right)\right]$	For each supply location j, sum up ratios r_i, discounted by distance decay function $f(d_{ij})$, across all demand locations i (=1, 2, ..., m), to yield crowdedness C_j at supply location j: $C_j = \sum_{i=1}^{m}\left[r_i f\left(d_{ij}\right)\right]$ $= \sum_{i=1}^{m}\left[D_i f\left(d_{ij}\right) / \sum_{l=1}^{n}\left(S_l f\left(d_{il}\right)\right)\right]$
Property	Weighted mean of accessibility (using the demand amount as weight) is equal to the ratio of total supply to total demand in the study area	Weighted mean of crowdedness (using the supply capacity as weight) is equal to the ratio of total demand to total supply in the study area
	Weighted means of accessibility and crowdedness are reciprocal of each other	

Revised from Wang (2021, p. 629).

best-fitting distance decay function is essential for reliable measures of accessibility for residents (or patients) and crowdedness for facilities.

3.3 Deriving the Distance Decay Functions by the Spatial Interaction Model

3.3.1 Estimating the Spatial Interaction Model

A simple *spatial interaction model*, or *gravity model*, is written as

$$T_{ij} = aO_iD_jf\left(d_{ij}\right) \tag{3.1}$$

where T_{ij} is the number of trips between area i and j, O_i is the size of an origin i (e.g., population in a residential area), D_j is the size of a destination j (e.g., hospital bed size), a is a scalar constant, and f is a function of the distance between i and j (denoted by d_{ij}). Note that both the origin size O_i and destination size D_j assume a unitary elasticity (exponent = 1) for simplicity.

Rearranging Equation 3.1 and taking logarithms on both sides yield

$$\ln I_{ij} = \ln\left(T_{ij} / \left(O_i D_j\right)\right) = \ln a + \ln f\left(d_{ij}\right)$$

Take the distance decay effect as a power function, $f\left(d_{ij}\right) = d_{ij}^{-\beta}$, for example. It becomes

$$\ln I_{ij} = A - \beta \ln d_{ij} \qquad (3.2)$$

where A is intercept $\ln a$, and β is the distance friction coefficient. The model can be estimated by a simple bivariate linear regression.

A similar logarithmic transformation can be applied to the other four distance decay functions, as summarized in Table 3.2. After their logarithmic transformations, all five functions can be estimated by a simple bivariate *linear ordinary least square (LOLS) regression*.

A more general spatial interaction model can be written as

$$T_{ij} = a O_i^{\alpha_1} D_j^{\alpha_2} f\left(d_{ij}\right) \qquad (3.3)$$

where α_1 and α_2 are the added exponents or elasticities for origin O_i and destination D_j, respectively.

Again, assuming a power function for the distance decay, the logarithmic transformation of Equation 3.3 is

$$\ln T_{ij} = \ln a + \alpha_1 \ln O_i + \alpha_2 \ln D_j - \beta \ln d_{ij} \qquad (3.4)$$

which can be estimated by a multivariate linear regression model.

TABLE 3.2

Distance Decay Functions and Log-Transforms for Regression

Distance Decay Function	Function Form	Log-Transform Used in Linear Regression	Restrictions
Power	$f(d) = d^{-\beta}$	$\ln I = A - \beta \ln d$	$I \neq 0$ and $d \neq 0$
Exponential	$f(d) = e^{-\beta d}$	$\ln I = A - \beta d$	$I \neq 0$
Square-root exponential	$f(d) = e^{-\beta \sqrt{d}}$	$\ln I = A - \beta \sqrt{d}$	$I \neq 0$
Normal	$f(d) = e^{-\beta d^2}$	$\ln I = A - \beta d^2$	$I \neq 0$
Log-normal	$f(d) = e^{-\beta (\ln d)^2}$	$\ln I = A - \beta (\ln d)^2$	$I \neq 0$ and $d \neq 0$

One may also use a *nonlinear least square (NLLS) regression* to derive Equation 3.1 or 3.3 directly. The results generally differ from those by the LOLS on the log-transformation (Equation 3.2 or 3.4) since the two have different dependent variables (T_{ij} in NLLS versus $\ln T_{ij}$ in LOLS) and imply different assumptions of the error term (Wang, 2015, p.123). The NLLS regression on T_{ij} weights all equal *absolute errors* equally, whereas the LOLS regression on $\ln T_{ij}$ weights all equal *percentage errors* equally. For example, for observations with large T_{ij} values, the LOLS scales down the contribution by their error terms by taking the logarithms. However, the NLLS places the same weight on the absolute errors, and thus those large T_{ij} values tend to exert a dominant effect on the regression result.

Both approaches are used in the literature, and the choice depends on the objective of a study, or often one's tolerance of technical complexity. Estimating the NLLS usually requires access to advanced statistical programs. Most use the LOLS for its easy implementation. Furthermore, a popular measure for an LOLS regression model's goodness of fit is R^2 (*coefficient of determination*), which is no longer applicable to the NLLS as the residuals from NLLS do not add up to 0. One may use a *pseudo-R^2* as an approximate measure of goodness of fit for NLLS.

Here, we use the sample data provided[1] to estimate the bivariate regressions listed in Table 3.2. Many gravity-based models assume a unitary elasticity for the effects of origins (e.g., residents) and destinations (e.g., facilities), such as the Huff model to be discussed in Chapter 5, the spatial accessibility measures (Wang, 2012), and the Garin–Lowry model (Wang, 2015, p. 219–221). By doing so, the distance friction coefficient derived from the best fitting function can be directly fed into these models.

To implement the five regressions in Table 3.2, an OD patient service flow table with 37,180 flows is compiled to include the following variables:

1. destination capacity D_j is defined as the staffed bed size for each of the 213 hospitals,

2. origin size O_i is defined as the population in each of the 983 ZIP code areas,

3. intensity of interaction T_{ij} is defined as the volume of patient service flow from each ZIP code area to each hospital (i.e., an OD pair), and

4. the corresponding travel time d_{ij} for each OD pair is defined as the drive time in minutes.

---

[1] Specifically, as outlined in Section 1.3, geodatabase FL _ HSA.gdb includes (1) a polygon feature class ZIP _ Code _ Area, (2) a point feature class Hosp _ ZIP, and (3) a stand-alone table OD _ All _ Flows, which are merged to form a dbase file OD _ All _ Flows.dbf as an input file for regression analysis.

The dependent variable in all five models is calibrated as $\ln I_{ij} = \ln\left(T_{ij}/\left(O_i D_j\right)\right)$, and the independent variable is various terms of d_{ij} such as $\ln d_{ij}$, d_{ij}, $\sqrt{d_{ij}}$, d_{ij}^2, and $\left(\ln d_{ij}\right)^2$.

One may refer to the SAS program Reg _ fitfunction.SAS included in the complimentary dataset to implement the regression analysis. The program (1) reads the data in DBF format (OD _ All _ Flows.dbf) with variables POPU, NUMBEDS, AllFlows, and Total _ Time that define O_i, D_j, T_{ij}, and d_{ij}, respectively; (2) extracts the non-zero records for $O_i>0$, $D_j>0$, and $T_{ij}>0$; (3) defines log-transformed variables; and (4) runs the five bivariate LOLS regression models and reports the results. Note that the program also includes an option to implement the NLLS regression on the power function.

For those without access to the SAS software, another program Reg _ fitfunction.R is included to fit the same regression models in R programming.

The regression results are reported in Table 3.3. The best-fitting distance decay function (with $R^2=0.4428$) is the power function, and its friction coefficient is 1.4343. This result will be used in the Huff model discussed in Chapter 5.

Figure 3.2 shows the scatter plot of $\ln I_{ij}$ and $\ln d_{ij}$ overlaid with the fitted power function (in log-transform) and demonstrates the power function as a good fit for the observations. Figure 3.3 shows the curves representing the five fitted distance decay functions.

3.3.2 Distance Decay Effects across Geographic Areas in Florida

This sub-section and Sub-section 3.4.2 are based on a recent study by Jia et al. (2019) that analyzes distance decay patterns of hospital inpatient visits in Florida, which used the same data source, i.e., the 2011 SID data in Florida, as most of the case studies in this book. This sub-section examines

TABLE 3.3

Regression Results on Distance Decay Functions by the Spatial Interaction Model

Distance Decay Function	n[a]	Intercept (A)	Friction Coefficient (β)	R^2
$\ln I = A - \beta \ln d$	37,180	−7.8397	1.4343	0.4428[b]
$\ln I = A - \beta d$	37,180	−12.7669	0.0145	0.2528
$\ln I = A - \beta\sqrt{d}$	37,180	−11.1968	0.2909	0.3557
$\ln I = A - \beta d^2$	37,180	−13.5965	0.000017	0.1064
$\ln I = A - \beta\left(\ln d\right)^2$	37,180	−10.7498	0.1670	0.4051

[a] Number of observations with $I\neq0$ and $d\neq0$.
[b] The best-fitting function in bold.

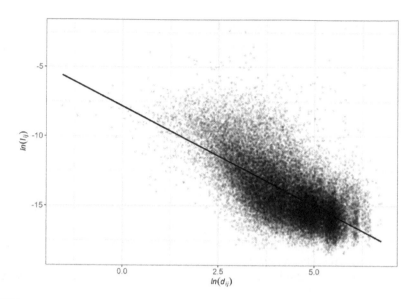

FIGURE 3.2
Scatter plot $\ln I_{ij}$ vs. $\ln d_{ij}$ overlaid with the fitted power function line.

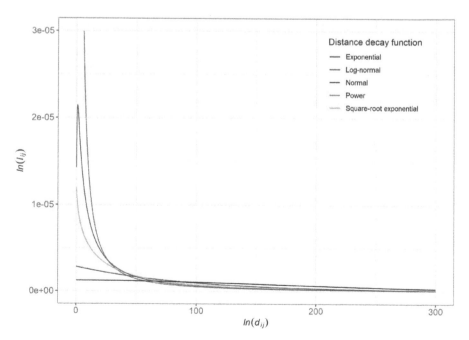

FIGURE 3.3
Fitted curves of five distance decay functions for all hospitalizations in Florida 2011.

the variability across geographic areas, where the best-fitting distance decay functions are derived by the spatial interaction model. Sub-section 3.4.2 explores the variability among subpopulations, where the best-fitting distance decay functions are derived by the complementary cumulative distribution curve approach.

The 2011 SID data in Florida contain individual records of patient discharge, and each record includes a range of individual socio-demographic factors of the patient, such as age, gender, race/ethnicity, and source of payment (e.g., health insurance type), ZIP codes of residence and hospital, and diagnostic information for the visit. For analysis on geographic areas in this sub-section, these individual records are aggregated to unique OD flows of patient service volumes from each ZIP code area to each hospital and then further divided into subsets by geographic areas. For analysis on population subgroups to be reported in Sub-section 3.4.2, those individual records are directly broken down to subsets by population subgroups. To further clarify the distinction in data preparation, the data subsets by geographic areas used in this sub-section are records of unique ZIP-to-hospital OD pairs with attributes such as ZIP code area population (origin size O_i), hospital bed size (destination capacity D_j), interaction intensity between them (volume of patient service flow T_{ij}), and corresponding travel time (drive time in minutes d_{ij}); and the data subsets by population groups used in Sub-section 3.4.2 remain individual records, only grouped to various socio-demographic groups and each record with corresponding travel time attached.

The study employs the more general form of spatial interaction model in Equation 3.3 to estimate distance decay effects. Three popular bivariate functions such as power, exponential, and normal (Gaussian) functions with one parameter β and the log-logistic function with two parameters α and β are tested. The log-logistic function cannot be linearized by log-transformation and thus cannot be estimated by LOLS. Therefore, the NLLS regression method is used for comparability of the four functions. In addition to pseudo-R^2, another index *Akaike information criterion (AIC)* is used to measure the performance of a regression. AIC measures the relative quality of the models due to varying complexities of four functions. A smaller AIC indicates a simpler model and is thus preferred.

The groupings of subsets are based on patients' ZIP code areas. First, all 983 ZIP codes are classified into four groups according to a national quartile classification by ZIP code median household income as follows: 1st (<\$39,000/year), 2nd (\$39,000–47,999), 3rd (\$48,000–62,999), and 4th (≥\$63,000). Next, the ZIP code areas are grouped into four urbanicity categories: large metropolitan (≥1 million residents), small metropolitan (50,000–1 million residents), micropolitan (10,000–49,999 residents), and rural areas. With only two exceptions where the exponential function has a slight edge, the log-logistic has the highest pseudo-R^2 and lowest AIC in all other subsets. Only the regression results by the log-logistic model are reported in Table 3.4. In the log-logistic

TABLE 3.4

Average Travel Time and Parameters in the Log-Logistic Function in the Spatial Interaction Model by Geographic Areas in Florida

	No. of Observations (n)	Average Travel Time (minutes)	α	β
All ZIP code areas	37,216	17.6	6.29	2.14
Median household income				
1st quartile	11,564	16.4	6.56	2.52
2nd quartile	10,339	17.7	6.53	2.14
3rd quartile	10,026	18.3	6.12	2.02
4th quartile	4,780	20.0	7.59	2.22
Urbanicity				
Large metropolitan	20,964	13.9	5.97	2.22
Small metropolitan	11,913	20.5	12.06	2.55
Micropolitan	2,894	34.2	14.53	3.20
Rural	1,445	50.9	11.20	1.82

function, the parameter $\alpha > 0$ is a scalar parameter, i.e., the median of the distribution, and the parameter $\beta > 0$ is a shape parameter. For a unimodal (one-hump) distribution with $\beta > 1$, a larger β corresponds to a distribution of less dispersion or steeper gradient and thus a stronger distance decay effect. In other words, a larger β indicates that more patients travel shorter and fewer patients travel longer for hospital visits. Table 3.4 also includes average travel time for each group of areas to give us some intuitive understanding of the travel burden in one area relative to others. As stated previously, the analytic function offers the whole spectrum of distribution across various travel ranges.

Based on the fitted functions in Table 3.4, Figures 3.4 and 3.5 illustrate various travel patterns across geographic areas of median household income ranges and across urbanicities, respectively. The curves are standardized by setting $O_i = 10,000$ and $D_j = 100$ to highlight the differing distance decay effects.

As shown in Figure 3.4, the distance decay gradient decreases from the 1st to 3rd quartile and ticks up in the 4th, consistent with the change of β reported in Table 3.4, implying a gradually decreasing distance decay effect before reaching the most affluent neighborhoods. The contrast between areas of the 1st and 4th quartiles is clear: A larger number of hospital visits occur within a short range (e.g., 16 minutes) from patient residences in the 1st quartile, but patient visits are much more spread out across travel time in the 4th quartile. Average travel time increases consistently from the 1st to 4th income levels. That is to say, patients from wealthier neighborhoods travel longer for hospital inpatient cares. On the one hand, the wealthier neighborhoods are usually farther away from hospitals, most of which are in downtown areas. On the other hand, patients from the neighborhoods of higher

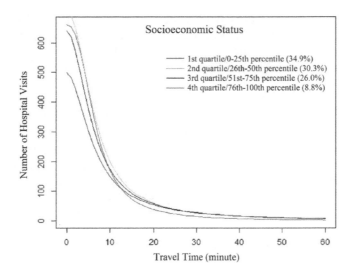

FIGURE 3.4
Log-logistic distance decay of patients across ZIP code median income groups in Florida 2011.

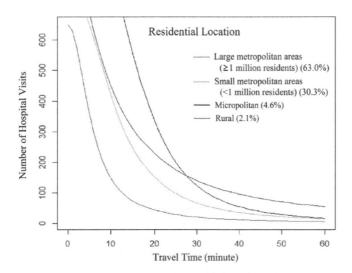

FIGURE 3.5
Log-logistic distance decay of patients across ZIP code urbanicity groups in Florida 2011.

average socioeconomic status tend to have better mobility and can afford traveling longer for better services. Here longer travel time for patients from more affluent neighborhoods does not necessarily reflect poorer accessibility, instead better mobility and perhaps preference of more choices in health care.

Note that the trend of β's change may not be completely consistent with that of average travel time. In this case, a declining β and thus a weakening distance decay effect from the 1st to 3rd quartile are consistent with a rising average travel time from the 1st to 3rd quartile. However, the distance decay parameter β ticks up and indicates a strengthening distance decay effect in the 4th quartile, but the average travel time continues to rise for this quartile. It seems counterintuitive for a stronger distance decay effect to correspond with a longer average travel time for patients in the 4th quartile. The reason lies in that the shape or distribution of the log-logistic function is jointly determined by the two parameters α and β. Here, as shown in Figure 3.4, a larger α value raises up the median of distribution while maintaining a steeper gradient β (or a more compressed shape in distribution), and the two counter each other (a larger α tends to drive up average travel time vs. a larger β tends to bring down average travel time) and result in a larger average travel time in the 4th quartile than in the 3rd quartile. In other words, the effect of the former dominates the latter. This further highlights the value of deriving a distance decay function to capture the distribution detail of travel time in place of a simply average travel time for an area here, and for a population group in Sub-section 3.4.2.

The vast majority of hospitals are located in metropolitan areas, with about two-thirds of hospitals in areas with a population of over 1 million. As reported in Table 3.4, the average travel time gradually increases with patients residing in less urbanized ZIP code areas, from large metropolitan (13.9 minutes) to small metropolitan (20.5 minutes), to micropolitan (34.2 minutes), and to rural areas (50.9 minutes). Both parameters α and β increase from large metropolitan to small metropolitan, and to micropolitan, but decrease in rural areas. That is to say, the median (captured by α) rises with a steepening gradient (β) from large metropolitan to small metropolitan, and to micropolitan, but the trend reverses in rural areas. This variability of distribution pattern across four types of urbanicities is well illustrated in Figure 3.5. In other words, hospitalizations in large metropolitan areas are highly concentrated in a short range (i.e., within 10 minutes from patients' residence) and the volume drops steeply toward longer trips. The curve moves higher while its gradient flattens in small metropolitan and further in micropolitan. In rural areas, the median (scalar) drops and the curve flattens. As discussed previously, the two counter each other and result in the longest travel time in rural areas. Here, the effect of flatter gradient in raising average travel time outpaces the effect of lower median in bringing down average travel time. To recap the distance decay effect, the number of hospital visits declines most rapidly with travel time in micropolitan areas ($\beta=3.20$), followed by small

(β=2.55) and then large metropolitan areas (β=2.22), and rural patients have the weakest distance decay effect (β=1.82). Most patients in small metropolitan areas spend 10–20 minutes traveling to hospitals, most micropolitan patients spend 15–30 minutes on traveling, and a larger proportion of rural patients spend ≥30 minutes on traveling than any other areas.

Obviously, rural patients travel longer for hospitalization as they are generally farther from their nearest hospitals than others. Furthermore, rural patients on average are much older, poorer, and sicker and have more complex health service needs that are only available in larger hospitals in major cities. This adds a major challenge for rural hospitals as they already suffer from a heavy loss of patients and revenue, have to cut back on services, and then are under more pressure to close (Sheps Center for Health Services Research, 2021).

3.4 Deriving the Distance Decay Functions by a Complementary Cumulative Distribution Curve

3.4.1 Estimating the Complementary Cumulative Distribution Function

In some studies, there are no data on measures of the attractions (sizes) of origins and destinations (O_i and D_j), and only the interaction intensity (e.g., patient service flow volume) between them (T_{ij}) is available. In that case, it is not feasible to define $I_{ij} = T_{ij} / (O_i D_j)$ and derive the distance decay function by the spatial interaction model. The *complementary cumulative distribution method* provides a solution. One may imagine that all origins are located at the center and the connected destinations are distributed in different rings by distance. The interaction intensity in the center is not measurable and often set as 1 when $d_{ij} = 0$. The outward interaction intensity gradually decreases and approaches zero with increasing distance from the center.

As shown in Figure 3.6, the percentage of patient volume increases up to 6 minutes for a corresponding band of estimated travel time (e.g., a 1-minute interval) and declines to near 0 when the travel time approaches 180 minutes. A complementary cumulative distribution is calibrated inversely from 180 to 0 minutes, where the cumulative percentage is near 0% at 180 minutes and increases to 100% at 0 minutes. In other words, the complementary cumulative percentage at any travel time is the percentage of patients who travel beyond that time. Various functions, similar to those outlined in Table 3.2, can be used to capture the distribution curve, and the best fitting one is identified by regressions.

As the travel time interval (band) varies, the complementary cumulative distribution pattern is largely consistent, and the parameters in the fitted

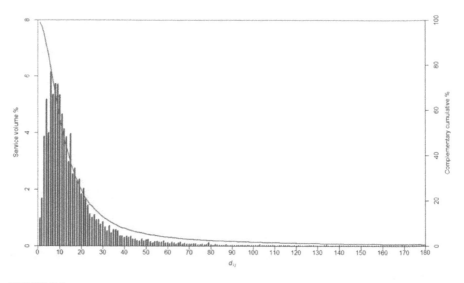

FIGURE 3.6
Service volume percentages and complementary cumulative percentages across travel time in minutes.

corresponding function change slightly. A larger interval leads to fewer observations for regression. For our case study, six travel time intervals ranging from 1 to 6 minutes are experimented, and among the five functions listed in Table 3.2, the power function yields the highest R^2 ranging from 0.8275 (1-minute interval) to 0.9386 (6-minute interval) across all six intervals. Table 3.5 reports the result when the travel time interval is 1 minute, and again shows that the power function is the best-fitting one.

The R program Reg _ ccdf.R is provided in the dataset to implement the process. The program (1) reads two variables AllFlows and Total _ Time from OD _ All _ Flows.dbf and extracts the non-zero records, (2) calculates the complementary cumulative probability for a given time interval, and (3) runs the five bivariate OLS regression models and reports the results.

3.4.2 Distance Decay Effects Across Population Groups in Florida

Different population groups may exhibit distinctive travel patterns for health care, here captured by differing distance decay functions. The differences may stem from their varying responses to spatial impedance to hospitals and also reflect the corresponding mobility and scopes of accessible health care choices. Also based on the study by Jia et al. (2019), this sub-section examines differential effects of distance decay on hospital inpatient visits among subpopulations in Florida. Much of the technical detail has been spelled out in the preceding sub-section. Here we focus on the findings and related implications.

TABLE 3.5

Regression Results on Distance Decay Functions by the
Complementary Cumulative Distribution Curve

Distance Decay Function	n^a	Intercept (A)	Friction Coefficient (β)	R^2
$\ln I = A - \beta \ln d$	**180**	**0.3306**	**0.9358**	**0.8275[b]**
$\ln I = A - \beta d$	180	−3.9704	0.0025	0.3824
$\ln I = A - \beta \sqrt{d}$	180	−2.8881	0.1111	0.5709
$\ln I = A - \beta d^2$	180	−4.544	0.000002	0.2306
$\ln I = A - \beta (\ln d)^2$	180	−2.0369	0.0885	0.7188

[a] Number of observations with 1-minute time interval.
[b] The best-fitting function in bold.

The subpopulations include breakdowns by age groups, genders, races/
ethnicities, and health insurance coverage. At least two reasons make it infeasible or unreliable to use the spatial interaction model to derive the distance
decay function. One is the lack of data for defining ZIP code area population
for each specific subgroup (origin size O_i) or hospital size dedicated/allocated
for that subgroup (destination capacity D_j). Another reason is that the patient
flow volumes T_{ij} between ZIP code areas and hospitals for specific subgroups
tend to be small values and make the statistical modeling based on the gravity model more sensitive to data errors. Therefore, the complementary cumulative distribution function is used to capture the distance decay effects of
hospital utilization in the subpopulations.

As trip length increases, the volume of patient services traveling beyond
that time declines, and the corresponding complementary percentage
becomes smaller. If a constant interval were used, the dependent variable
(complementary percentage) would be less reliable (e.g., more sensitive to
data or estimation errors) for long travel time[2]. Specifically, this study defines
the data points as follows:

1. one for every minute for the range [0, 30 minutes] (31 points),
2. one for every 5 minutes for the range (30, 60 minutes] (6 points),
3. one for every 10 minutes for (60, 120 minutes) (5 points), and
4. the data point at 120 minutes includes all patient volumes beyond
   120 minutes (1 point).

---

[2] In the illustrative example in Sub-section 3.4.1, all patients are grouped together without
breaking down to subgroups and a constant travel time interval is used since the sample size
is sufficient across all intervals.

This yields a total number of observations $n=31+6+5+1=43$ for the overall model and each subgroup, reported in Table 3.6.

Similarly, the NLLS regression is used to estimate the parameters. Based on the regression results such as *pseudo*-R^2 and AIC values (not reported here, see Jia et al. (2019) for details), the log-logistic function produces the best fit with a *pseudo*-R^2 as high as 0.9999. A good fit for regression by the complementary

TABLE 3.6

Average Travel Time and Parameters in the Log-Logistic Function by the Complementary Cumulative Distribution Function by Subpopulations in Florida

	No. of Patients	Average Travel Time (minutes)	n^a	α	β
Overall	2,376,743	17.6	43	10.725	1.870
Age					
<12	278,094	19.8	43	13.332	2.056
<12 (no newborn)	75,696	26.3	43	15.566	1.769
12–17	35,232	25.3	43	15.387	1.852
18–24	126,525	19.4	43	11.573	1.912
25–34	222,157	18.2	43	11.912	2.011
35–44	190,860	18.5	43	11.211	1.892
45–54	273,250	18.2	43	10.437	1.788
55–64	313,738	18.6	43	10.577	1.789
65–74	353,623	18.1	43	10.602	1.817
≥75	583,227	14.3	43	8.993	1.933
Gender					
Male	1,026,589	18.3	43	10.695	1.790
Female	1,350,140	17.1	43	10.710	1.914
Race/Ethnicity					
White	1,489,589	19.2	43	11.528	1.809
Black	400,428	14.7	43	9.152	2.027
Hispanic	399,395	14.0	43	9.540	2.089
Asian	19,837	16.7	43	11.526	2.263
Native	3,343	23.9	43	12.208	1.631
Others	41,976	21.3	43	13.032	1.964
Health Insurance					
Medicare	1,074,328	16.0	43	9.632	1.867
Medicaid	498,513	17.6	43	11.055	1.896
Private	531,698	20.8	43	12.987	1.977
Self-pay	144,432	17.5	43	9.951	1.797
No-charge	45,300	12.6	43	8.641	2.146

[a] Number of observations with 1-minute interval for [0, 30 minutes], 5-minute interval for (30, 60 minutes], 10-minute interval for (60, 120 minutes), and 1 observation for >=120 minutes.

cumulative probability approach is common since the values on the y-axis are cumulative and monotonically decline. A study by Delamater et al. (2013) also reports an excellent curve fit by the same function.

As shown in Table 3.6, with increasing age of patients, the parameter α and thus the median value of distribution generally declines: The younger groups (age <18) have $\alpha > 13$, groups with age 18–44 have α ranging 11–12, groups with age 45–74 have α around 10.5, and the elderly (age ≥75) has the lowest $\alpha < 9$. This is consistent with the trend of declining average travel time to hospitals with increasing age. The trend for the parameter β characterizing the shape of distribution is less clear. A more compressed pattern (a steeper declining gradient) is observed for the age groups of the youngest (<12), the oldest (≥75), and the middle (25–34). The difference between genders in distance decay behavior is negligible, both in terms of average travel time and in terms of the derived distance decay functions.

The variabilities across racial-ethnic groups and health insurance carriers are of great interest in many health studies. Due to relatively small numbers of discharge records for Asians and Native Americans, results from the derived distance decay functions for these two subgroups may not be very reliable, and hence our discussion on them is limited to that based on the average travel time. Native Americans travel the longest time on average (23.9 minutes) for hospitalization services, possibly due to a disproportionally high number of them residing in remote rural areas in Florida. Whites spend the second longest travel time to hospitals on average (19.2 minutes), followed by Asians (16.7 minutes), Blacks (14.7 minutes), and Hispanics (14.0 minutes). Figure 3.7 depicts the distribution patterns of distance decay

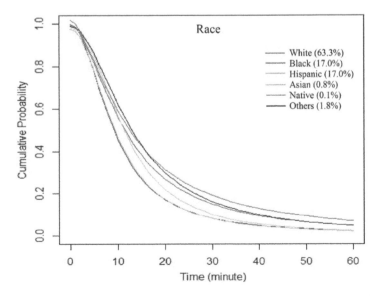

FIGURE 3.7
Log-logistic distance decay of patients across racial/ethnic groups in Florida 2011.

effects across the racial-ethnic groups. Blacks and Hispanics have a similar hospital utilization pattern with similar values in parameters α and β. The median parameter α is significantly higher for Whites than for Blacks and Hispanics, consistent with a higher average travel time for Whites, and the shape parameter β is smaller for Whites than for Blacks and Hispanics, indicating a weaker distance decay effect (or a flatter gradient and a pattern of more dispersion) for Whites. The contrast is evident in Figure 3.7 that shows a considerable portion (>20%) of Whites travelling beyond 30 minutes and less than 20% Blacks or Hispanics going beyond 20 minutes.

Figure 3.8 shows the distribution patterns for patients paid by different (or lack of) health insurance plans for hospital services. The major contrast is between the no-charge patients (those discharged without paying) and privately insured. The former has the lowest α (8.641), and the latter the highest α (12.987), consistent with the shortest average travel time (12.6 minutes) and the longest average travel time (20.8 minutes) observed, respectively. The no-charge patients also have the largest β value, i.e., the strongest distance decay effect, and thus are highly concentrated in short-range trips. Following the no-charge group, Medicare beneficiaries spend the second shortest average time (16.0 minutes), followed by self-pay patients (17.5 minutes), Medicaid beneficiaries (17.6 minutes), and finally the privately insured (20.8 minutes). Once again, the order of average travel time is consistent with the order of α. The value of β is the highest (indicating the largest gradient or the most compressed distribution) for the no-charge group, and declines further in the order of privately insured, Medicaid beneficiaries, Medicare beneficiaries, and self-pay patients, reflecting an increasing dispersion in travel ranges.

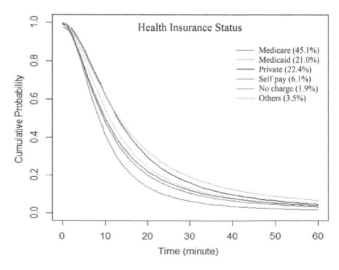

FIGURE 3.8
Log-logistic distance decay of patients across payment groups in Florida 2011.

The comparison among racial-ethnic subgroups reveals that the mobility for seeking hospital services is more limited for Blacks and Hispanics than for Whites. The longest average travel time by Native Americans sends an alarm and highlights the challenge of accessibility for this group that is highly concentrated in remote rural areas (Lester, 1999). Further research using datasets with larger numbers of Native Americans and Asians is needed to better reveal their travel patterns for hospital visits. The results about travel behavior across health insurance coverages reinforce some previous findings that patients covered by private insurance or managed care plans are more likely to bypass local hospitals and travel longer for hospitalization than Medicare and Medicaid beneficiaries and the uninsured (e.g., self-pay and no-charge patients) (Radcliff et al., 2003; Escarce and Kapur, 2009). The racial-ethnic variable also intersects with the health insurance carrier variable. For example, Blacks and Hispanics are significantly more likely than Whites to be uninsured. Examining such an intersection requires access to data of large populations that can be further divided into more-detailed population subgroups while maintaining sufficient sample sizes.

3.5 Summary

This chapter examined the spatial behavior of patients in health care utilization through the lens of distance decay. A distance decay function is an analytical way to capture the whole spectrum of patients traveling different distances for seeking health care and is thus a more comprehensive and yet elegant way (e.g., with a single distance friction coefficient) to reflect their spatial behavior than traditionally used average travel distance. For example, a flatter gradient in a distance decay function usually corresponds to a longer range of travel on average. Like two sides of the same coin, a longer range in seeking cares by a group indicates more travel burden and thus a disadvantaged location for the group; in the meantime, it may also indicate a group with higher mobility and being more selective in health cares received (e.g., bypassing closer providers for more distant and perhaps higher-quality services). One may relate it to the paradox of residential choice as city dwellers balance proximity to jobs for saving in commuting versus more spacious housing. As a result, average commuting range tends to increase with income, but the highest income earners retreat to shorter commutes (Wang, 2003).

Among commonly used forms, the power, exponential, square-root exponential, Gaussian, and log-normal functions have only one parameter, termed "distance friction coefficient". More complicated forms such as the log-logistic and compound power-exponential functions have two or more parameters. Deriving and analyzing the best-fitting distance decay function is a valuable endeavor in health care studies. First, it helps solidify the theoretical foundation of a hierarchal structure in health care market, where the smaller and more HSAs are anchored by general hospitals and larger and fewer HRRs are led by specialized hospitals. Patients for the former experience distance decay with a steeper gradient. Second, the derived distance decay function is an important component in models that are built upon the spatial interactions between residents and hospitals (e.g., the Huff model in Chapter 5). Third, the function may also help improve some algorithms in network community detection and potentially benefit the research on HSA delineation by that approach (Chapter 6).

The distance decay functions can be estimated by a spatial interaction model, where the service volumes are positively related to the sizes of origins (residential areas) and destinations (hospitals) and reversely related to the distances between them. For the aforementioned five one-parameter functions, the best-fitting model can be empirically derived by linear ordinary least square (LOLS) regression on their logarithmic transformations, or nonlinear least square (NLLS) regression on their original forms. In the absence of data on the sizes of origins and destinations, the distance decay functions can be estimated by the complementary cumulative distribution function method. It simply displays how the inversely cumulative percentages of service volumes (i.e., the percentage of patients who travel beyond a range) decline with distances. The same set of functions can be used to fit the curve.

The case study in Florida uses the best-fitting distance decay functions derived by the spatial interaction model to examine the variability across geographic areas, and those derived by the complementary cumulative distribution function method to examine the variability across population groups. In both cases, the log-logistic function produces the best fit. By geographic areas, patients spend longer travel time to hospitals on average as the urbanicity level of their residence decreases from large metropolitan to small metropolitan, micropolitan, and rural areas, and the distance decay effect weakens in wealthier neighborhoods. Across population groups, distance decay effects generally increase with patient ages; Whites spend the longest travel time to hospitals on average, followed by Asians, Blacks, and Hispanics; and no-charge patients spend the shortest travel time to hospitals on average, followed by Medicare beneficiaries, self-pay patients, Medicaid beneficiaries, and the privately insured.

4

Delineating Hospital Service Areas by the Dartmouth Method

The most popular units for analysis of geographic variability of health care market are the hospital service areas (HSAs) and hospital referral regions (HRRs) developed by the Dartmouth Atlas of Health Care Project. HSAs and HRRs represent the local health care market for inpatient care and tertiary medical care, respectively. An HRR is composed of at least one HSA, usually several whole HSAs, and thus HRR is a larger and a higher level of unit than HSA. There were 3,436 HSAs and 306 HRRs defined by the Dartmouth Atlas of Health Care Project in 1993. Both units are constructed to capture the most interactions between patients and service providers and offer reliable analysis units for the assessment of health care market.

This chapter discusses the Dartmouth method as a foundation for other methods to be built upon and compare. Section 4.1 reviews the history of Dartmouth HSAs and HRRs, types of health care service areas developed by the method, and applications. Section 4.2 outlines the algorithms for defining HSAs and HRRs by the Dartmouth method, identifies challenges, and introduces the refined Dartmouth method so that it can be replicated consistently. Section 4.3 introduces an automated toolkit, composed of multiple tools, for implementing the refined Dartmouth method. Section 4.4 uses a case study to illustrate the implementations of defining HSAs and HRRs in Florida and evaluates the derived units. Section 4.5 concludes the chapter with a summary.

4.1 History and Applications of Dartmouth HSAs and HRRs

The *Dartmouth Atlas of Health Care Project* began in 1993 to study the geographic variations of health care resources and their utilization in the USA (www.dartmouthatlas.org). For small area analysis and mapping, administrative units below the state level (e.g., county or city) do not necessarily capture health care markets, so the Project piloted the delineations of HSAs and HRRs as analysis units for local hospital market areas and tertiary areas, respectively. The Medicare data, while limited to patients of 65 years or older, from a single payer Centers for Medicare and Medicaid Services (CMS), became a natural choice for a nationwide study. While the annual reports

DOI: 10.1201/9780429260285-4

are available from 1994 onward, the HSAs and HRRs derived from the 1993 Medicare data have remained largely intact over the years.

The Dartmouth Atlas of Health Care Project has also used the same method to develop other specific service areas. For example, the *pediatric surgical areas (PSAs)* are defined for the Northern New England by aggregating HSAs based on children's travel for common ENT procedures and appendectomies. The *primary care service areas (PCSAs)* are based on Medicare patients for primary care providers in the USA. In terms of impacts, none comes close to the wide usage of Dartmouth HSAs and HRRs, which are the focus of this chapter.

There is a large body of literature that examines the magnitude and underlying causes of geographic variations in health care supply, access, utilization, spending, outcomes, and their associations with other socio-demographic factors across the Dartmouth HSAs and HRRs. For instance, Goodman and Fisher (2008) evaluated the supply of physicians across HRRs to illustrate the essence of physician workforce crisis in the USA. An influential Dartmouth report on the variability of end-of-life cancer care costs for Medicare beneficiaries was also based on the HRRs (Goodman et al., 2010). Radley and Schoen (2012) examined the variation in access to care and its association with quality of health care received across HRRs and suggested that improving access and care quality takes collaborative efforts from multiple stakeholders such as local physicians, insurance companies, and policymakers. Understandably, most of these studies at the national scale relied on the HRRs as the number of HRRs (306) was manageable.

However, HRRs are fairly large with a minimum population of 120,000. In order to gain a better resolution, one needs to use HSAs. Because of its large number (3,436) in the entire USA, studies on the variability across HSAs are more likely to limit their scope to a state or a region. For example, Ward et al. (2014) examined how access to oncologists affected chemotherapies received by cancer patients across the HSAs in Iowa. A notable study by Zhang et al. (2012) highlighted the importance of using HSAs in place of HRRs in explaining the variability of Medicare costs across the USA. They found that about 41% of the variation in adjusted HSA drug spending was between HRRs and the remaining 59% was within HRRs. Implication of the study calls for policies to target HSAs instead of HRRs. Another study by Rosenberg et al. (2016) used the data from the Healthcare Cost and Utilization Project (HCUP, covers regions of about 50% of the US population) to explain the variabilities of inpatient mortality, inpatient safety, and prevention outcomes and found significant variabilities at both the HSA and HRR levels.

These studies certainly demonstrate the value of HSAs and HRRs in analyzing geographic disparities in health care and shedding light on policy reform. In the meantime, it is just as important to ensure the reliability and validity of these two geographic units.

There are at least three reasons to update and refine the Dartmouth HSAs and HRRs. First, the 1992–1993 Medicare data used for the definitions are outdated. The health care market has experienced major changes such as hospital closures, expansion, new openings, and consolidation. Some HSAs no longer contain any hospitals. Second, the Medicare data only cover the population of 65 years or older that were enrolled in the program and may not represent the general population. The units may be biased toward the ill beneficiaries who use disproportionally more inpatient or tertiary care than other age groups. Thirdly, the methods for deriving HSAs and HRRs involve uncertainties with limited automation. For example, visual examination of preliminary results is required to ensure spatial contiguity for HSAs or HRRs, and subsequent decisions are made manually. The process is also time-consuming and even cost prohibitive for timely update. This may help explain the lack of updates on the Dartmouth HSAs and HRRs and is a major motivation for us to develop an automated tool that can be replicated on a consistent basis.

4.2 The Dartmouth Method for Defining HSAs and HRRs

4.2.1 Defining HSAs by the Refined Dartmouth Method

According to the Dartmouth Atlas of Health Care Project, prepared by the Center for Evaluative Clinical Sciences (1999), the Dartmouth method defines HSAs in three steps:

1. All acute care hospitals identified from the American Hospital Association and the Medicare provider files are assigned to the town or city in which they are located to form candidate HSAs ($N=3,953$). An HSA is named after the town or city.

2. All hospitalization records are aggregated from each ZIP code area of patients to each hospital. For "point ZIP codes" (specific institutions or PO Box), they are assigned to the enclosing ZIP code areas. If a town or city has multiple hospitals, the records are combined. A *plurality rule* is applied to assign each ZIP code area to the HSA, with which the hospitals are most often used.

3. The ZIP codes being assigned to the hospitals in the same town would form an HSA. The HSAs are examined visually and adjusted to ensure all HSAs are geographically contiguous.

The three-step Dartmouth method seemed straightforward and yielded 3,436 HSAs based on 1992–1993 Medicare data.

However, each step encounters some complexity or uncertainty to be resolved:

1. In step 1, some cities (e.g., New York, Los Angeles, Chicago, and Houston) are very large with multi-million population. If one city with any number of hospitals forms one candidate HSA, the HSAs in those large cities would be too large to reflect local hospital markets.

Our research on the database of Dartmouth HSAs reveals multiple HSAs in each of those cities; however, the document does not clarify how a large city is divided. Here, it is termed *"the large city problem"*.

2. In step 2, after applying the plurality rule, a significant number (about 500) of candidate HSAs have more patients living in those HSAs that are hospitalized in other HSAs. In other words, a ZIP code area with at least a hospital being visited most often by other ZIP code area(s) sends the largest volume of patients to another ZIP code area. According to the Dartmouth Atlas of Health Care Project, these candidate HSAs are considered not independent. It is termed *"the non-independent HSA problem"*.

3. Also, in step 2, how to define the most hospitalization between a ZIP code and an HSA is not clarified. The most hospitalization can be the sum of all hospitalization between a ZIP code and all ZIP codes in one HSA or the maximum hospitalization between the ZIP code and another ZIP code in one HSA. It is termed *"the maximum hospitalization problem"*.

4. In step 3, the document shows that an island ZIP code is reassigned to the enclosing HSA and provides an example of assigning an enclaved ZIP code to its neighboring HSA. However, it does not provide systematic rules to process these spatially non-contiguous HSAs. We term it *"the spatial non-contiguity problem"*.

The above four problems need to be addressed in order to implement the Dartmouth method for delineating HSAs consistently and reliably.

One important task for updating the Dartmouth method is to derive a spatial adjacency matrix between ZIP code areas for identifying contiguous HSAs. A spatial adjacency matrix may be defined in two ways: (1) Rook contiguity defines adjacent areas as those sharing edges, and (2) queen contiguity defines adjacent areas as those sharing edges or nodes (Cliff and Ord, 1973). For our purpose, the queen contiguity is used. The row and column in the spatial adjacency matrix are identified by an origin ZIP code area and a destination ZIP code area, respectively. If two ZIP code areas are adjacent, the value in the corresponding row and column is 1, and 0 otherwise. The matrix also needs to account for two scenarios. One involves the ZIP code areas off the coast. They are geographic islands, but are connected to the mainland by bridges, ferry boats, or other means. A link like a virtual bridge is built, coded 1 in the spatial adjacency matrix, to connect a ZIP code area in the island and another ZIP code area in the mainland that has the shortest distance between them. In the second scenario, some ZIP code areas are separated by natural barriers, such as rivers, wildlife management areas, or parks. They are connected via physical roads, bridges, or ferryboats. One may need to examine local geography (e.g., via Google Maps) to validate the connection and adjust the spatial adjacency matrix accordingly.

Figure 4.1 shows a snapshot of seven ZIP code areas: each labeled with ZoneID-1 ranging from 665 to 671 on the left side and the corresponding

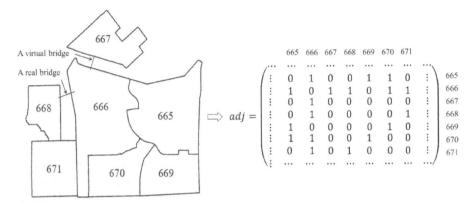

FIGURE 4.1
Building a spatial adjacency matrix for ZIP code areas.

spatial adjacency matrix on the right side. Since the value of ZoneID starts from 1, the symmetric matrix has each row and column represented by ZoneID-1 starting from 0 in the programming tool. For example, the ZIP code labeled with 666 shares the edges with the ZIP codes labeled with 665, 670, and 671 based on the queen contiguity, so their corresponding values are 1 in the matrix. In addition, the geographic island, ZIP code labeled with 667 in one cluster, is connected to the nearest ZIP code labeled with 666 in another cluster by a virtual bridge, so that their corresponding values are 1 in the matrix as well. The ZIP code labeled with 668 is connected to the ZIP code labeled with 666 with a physical bridge (road), so their corresponding values are also 1 in the matrix. Note that the spatial adjacency matrix has the diagonal values of 0 to code the relationship from a ZIP code area to itself.

Using the spatial adjacency matrix and the ZIP-to-ZIP network of hospitalization, we update and implement the Dartmouth method for defining HSAs in three steps:

1. Identify each unique destination ZIP code area from the network of hospitalization to anchor the initial HSA instead of a city or town. This solves "the large city problem".

2. Assign a ZIP code area to an HSA with the highest service volume among other destination HSAs, and ensure that the HSA is also spatially adjacent to that ZIP code area. If the ZIP code has hospitalization flows to multiple ZIP codes in the same HSA, add up the flows together before assessing the maximum one. It solves the "maximum hospitalization problem". If the flows are tied as the maximum, assign the ZIP code to the HSA with the smallest population for most gain in balancing region size. If the ZIP code has the maximum flow going to a non-adjacent HSA, leave it unassigned for next iteration. When a ZIP code is assigned to an HSA whose maximum

flow goes to another adjacent HSA, they are non-independent HSAs. The rule calls for merging all non-independent HSAs to solve "the non-independent HSA problem".

3. Repeat step 2 until all ZIP code areas are assigned to the adjacent HSA. If the ZIP code has no patients going to its adjacent HSAs, assign it to the HSA with the smallest population and at least one hospital for most gain in balancing region size. This solves "the spatial non-contiguity problem".

Both patients and hospitals are consolidated into ZIP code areas so that each node represents the ZIP code of patients or the ZIP code of hospitals or both. Edge weight is service flow volume from a ZIP code of patients to a ZIP code of hospitals, and thus it is a directed weighted network. The network optimization method introduced in Chapter 6 deals with an undirected weighted network.

Figure 4.2 illustrates the implementation of the refined Dartmouth method for defining HSAs with graphs on the left and corresponding explanations on the right. The illustrative example has nine nodes (ZIP code areas) indexed as 1–9 in circles. The solid lines labeled with numbers refer to the

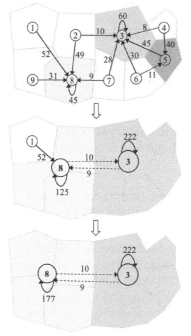

Step 1: identify three initial HSAs: HSA (3), HSA (5), and HSA (8)
Step 2:
1. first iteration to assign ZIP code to adjacent HSA:
   • assign 1 to 8 (max flows = 52), not adjacent, retain 1
   • assign 2 to 8 (max flows = 49) -> HSA (2,8)
   • assign 3 to 3 (max flows = 60) -> HSA (3)
   • assign 4 to 5 (max flows = 40) -> HSA (4,5)
   • assign 5 to 3 (max flows = 45) -> HSA (3,4,5)
   • assign 6 to 3 (max flows = 30+11) -> HSA (3,4,5,6)
   • assign 7 to 3 (max flows = 28) -> HSA (3,4,5,6,7)
   • assign 8 to 8 (max flows = 45) -> HSA (2,8)
   • assign 9 to 8 (max flows = 31) -> HSA (2,8,9)

   ❖ generate two HSAs, HSA (8) and HSA (3) that contains ZIP codes (2,8,9) and (3,4,5,6,7),
   ❖ aggregate edge flows between ZIP codes and HSAs.

2. second iteration to assign ZIP code to adjacent HSA:
   • assign 1 to 8 (max flows = 52) -> HSA (1,8)

   ❖ generate two HSAs, HSA (8) and HSA (3) that contains ZIP codes (1,2,8,9) and (3,4,6,7),
   ❖ aggregate edge flows between HSAs and HSAs.

Step 3: all ZIP codes are assigned.
   ❖ generate **two HSAs**: HSA (8) and HSA (3),
      • contains ZIP codes (1,2,8,9) and (3,4,5,6,7), respectively,
      • contains 1 and 2 hospitals, respectively.

① ② ◌ ⑧ ZIP codes or HSAs   ZIP code areas represent locations of patients or hospitals   HSAs

⟶ Flows from a ZIP code of patients to a ZIP code of hospitals   ┈┈➤ Flows between HSAs via ZIP codes of patients

FIGURE 4.2
Schematic illustration of the refined Dartmouth method for delineating HSAs.

service flow volumes with arrows pointing from the ZIP code of patients to the ZIP code of hospitals, including two self-loops (nodes 3 and 8) with patients visiting hospitals within the same ZIP code areas. Step 1 identifies three destination ZIP codes with hospitals as three initial HSAs: HSA(3), HSA(5), and HSA(8). Step 2 has two iterations to assign each ZIP code to the adjacent HSA connected by the highest service volume. The first iteration initially assigns nodes 2, 8, and 9 to HSA(8); nodes 3, 5, 6, and 7 to HSA(3); and node 4 to HSA(5). As node 1 goes to a non-adjacent HSA(8) with the highest volume, it is unassigned at this stage. Node 4 goes to HSA(5), which goes to HSA(3), and according to the rule for consolidating the "non-independent HSAs", HSA(5) is merged to HSA(3), which now contains five nodes (3, 4, 5, 6, and 7). The second iteration finds node 1 unassigned and is then assigned to the expanded HSA(8) composed of three ZIP code areas (2, 8, and 9), which becomes adjacent to node 1. Step 3 ends by verifying that all nodes have been assigned, forming two final HSAs: HSA(8) contains four nodes (1, 2, 8, and 9) and HSA(3) contains five nodes (3, 4, 5, 6, and 7).

For defining HSAs, two optional rules may be considered whether either or both are desirable: (1) each HSA with a minimum population, such as 1,000 as suggested in defining the primary care service areas (PCSAs) (Goodman et al., 2003) and (2) each HSA with a minimum localization index (LI), e.g., 0.5, used in some existing studies (Jia et al., 2017b; Haynes, Wertli, and Aujesky, 2020). LI refers to the proportion of patients that receive services in hospitals within an HSA out of total patients from the HSA.

The refined Dartmouth method clarifies, for the first time, three important processes in step 2, highlighted in dash rectangles in Figure 4.2, which were not clarified in the original Dartmouth method. The first one is the definition of the adjacent HSAs with the highest service volumes. Node 1 has the largest service volume (52) to the non-adjacent HSA(8) so that it is unassigned in the first iteration and eventually assigned to it in the second iteration after the expanded HSA becomes adjacent to it. The second one refers to the non-independent HSA problem. Node 4 is initially assigned to the adjacent HSA(5), whose maximum flow volume (=45) goes to its adjacent HSA(3). The two non-independent HSAs are merged. The third one illustrates the process of updating edge weights (flows) between HSAs, which also refers to the maximum hospitalization problem. For example, after merging nodes 3, 4, and 5 to form HSA(3), the flow from node 6 to HSA(3) is the sum of flows from node 6 to all member nodes of HSA(3), i.e., 41 (=30+11).

4.2.2 Defining HRRs by the Refined Dartmouth Method

The HRRs defined by the Dartmouth Atlas Project in 1993 were constructed from a total of 3,436 HSAs in the USA. There are also three steps:

1. Candidate HSAs are identified as those performing at least ten major cardiovascular surgical procedures (DRGs 103–107) and at least one specified major neurosurgical procedure (DRGs 1–3 and 484) on

Medicare enrollees for 2 years (1992–1993). Candidate HSAs form initial HRRs ($N=458$).

2. Each HSA is assigned to the initial HRRs by applying the plurality rule based on the major cardiovascular surgical procedures and neurosurgery.

3. The above provisional HRRs are further adjusted according to three rules: (1) geographic contiguity (with exceptions justified by, for example, separation by major travel routes), (2) a threshold population size of 120,000, and (3) a threshold LI, e.g., 0.65.

The three-step Dartmouth method yielded 306 HRRs based on the 1992–1993 Medicare data.

Similar uncertainties also apply to the delineation of Dartmouth HRRs and call for refinements in order to replicate the method on a consistent basis. Two data preparation tasks also proceed the method's implementation: aggregating the ZIP-to-ZIP network of cardiovascular surgery and neurosurgery service flows to an HSA-to-HSA network, and deriving a spatial adjacency matrix for the HSA layer. After that, the refined Dartmouth method for defining HRRs is implemented in three steps:

1. Identify unique destination HSAs as initial HRRs, which form the maximum number of HRRs.

2. Assign each HSA to an adjacent HRR where the highest volume of patients from that HSA went for cardiovascular surgery and neurosurgery, and repeat the step until all HSAs are assigned. The same strategy outlined in step 2 of defining HSAs is adopted here to address "the non-independent HRR problem".

3. Assign each of the remaining HSAs to its adjacent HRR with the maximum cardiovascular surgery and neurosurgery flow volume. The same strategy in step 3 of defining HSAs is applied here to address possible "spatially non-contiguous HRRs" and ensure each HRR contains at least one specialized hospital where the two surgery services were performed.

Two additional rules are established in step 3 for defining HRRs: (1) the threshold population of 120,000 and (2) the minimum LI of 0.65. Most likely, the original Dartmouth method enforced both rules. Here, our refined method offers the options of enforcing them separately or jointly in delineating HRRs so that we will have a chance to evaluate their impacts. Assign the HRR to its adjacent HRR with the highest service volume of cardiovascular surgery and neurosurgery until the chosen criterion is (criteria are) met. If there is no service volume to any adjacent HRRs, assign it to the smallest one with maximum gain in balancing region size.

Figure 4.3 shows how the delineations of HSAs and HRRs by the refined Dartmouth method differ. Foremost, HSAs are constructed of ZIP code areas

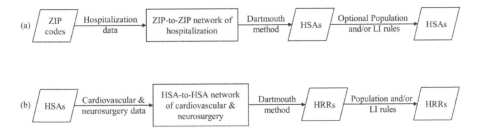

FIGURE 4.3
Defining (a) HSAs from ZIP code areas and (b) HRRs from HSAs.

by utilizing the hospitalization flow network between ZIP code areas, whereas HRRs are made of whole newly constructed HSAs by utilizing the network of cardiovascular surgery and neurosurgery flows between HSAs. In addition, constraints such as threshold values for population size and/or LI are added by us as an option for defining HSAs (e.g., experimenting with minimum population = 1,000 and/or minimum LI = 0.5), but are enforced in defining HRRs (i.e., minimum population = 120,000 and/or minimum LI = 0.65).

The Dartmouth method uses cardiovascular surgery and neurosurgery as the specialized hospital care to characterize the higher level (tertiary) care for hospitals in defining HRRs and uses all hospitalization (inpatient) care to characterize the basic (general) care for hospitals in defining HSAs. Recent studies such as Hu et al. (2018) indicate that the network structure of cardiac and neurosurgery service flows increasingly resembles that of all hospitalizations due to the rising availability and prevalence of these surgeries in the US hospitals. The number of these specialized hospitals ($N=192$) is also close to the number of all hospitals ($N=213$) in Florida. This may suggest the need of revisiting the use of these two services in defining the HRRs. In the next two sections, we explore the option of using neurosurgery alone, in addition to the combined cardiac and neurosurgery, as the specialized hospital care for defining HRRs.

4.3 Automating the Refined Dartmouth Method for HSA & HRR Delineations

The automation of the refined Dartmouth method is implemented in a toolkit of "HSA Delineation Pro.tbx".

Before using the toolkit, we suggest all layers and tables be saved in a geodatabase to avoid truncated field names that may not be identified by the tools. The following Python packages also need to be installed:

1. SciPy is a free and open-source Python library used for scientific and technical computing of mathematics, science, and engineering. It is released under the New BSD License (https://www.scipy.org/).

2. NetworkX is also a free Python library for creating, manipulating, and studying the structure and functions of complex networks, including graphs, digraphs, and multigraphs. It is released under the New BSD License (https://networkx.org/).

3. The igraph package is a collection of network analysis tools for creating, manipulating, analyzing, and visualizing networks. It is implemented in C and extended to Python and R versions (https://igraph.org/). It is released under the GNU GPL2 license. The NetworkX and igraph packages are both developed for network analysis.

4. The leidenalg package is free and developed by Traag et al. (2019) for implementing Leiden and Louvain algorithms. It is released under the GNU GPL2 v3.0 license.

To install four packages, users need to create or clone a Python environment as the default arcgispro-py3 in ArcGIS Pro is read-only and is not recommended to be modified to avoid unintended consequences. In ArcGIS Pro, click the Project tab and click Python to access the Python Package Manager. Click the Manage Environments button to open the dialog window, click the Clone Default button to clone the default environment, and name it (e.g., `arcgispro-py3-clone`). It may take a while to install all default packages. After that, the cloned environment is created in the folder `%LocalAppData%\Esri\conda\envs`. For example, in our case, it is under C:\Users\wang\AppData\Local\ESRI\conda\envs\arcgispro-py3-clone. Click OK to close the dialog window, and restart ArcGIS Pro[1].

Right-click the Start Menu button at the left end of the taskbar, select Run to launch the Run command window, enter cmd in the Open, and click OK to open the command prompt window.

- Type "cd C:\Users\wang\AppData\Local\ESRI\conda\envs\arcgispro-py3-clone" (in our case), and press Enter on the keyboard to go to the clone environment.

- Use the provided `requirements.txt` file under the data folder, for example, in D disk. Type "python -m pip install -r D:\Florida\requirements.txt" to install four packages simultaneously.

In ArcGIS Pro, under Catalog view, right-click Toolboxes and click Add Toolbox to open the dialog window. Select and add the "HSA Delineation" toolkit from the folder `Florida`. Expand the toolkit to display five tools:

1. Build a spatial adjacency matrix,[2] shown in Figure 4.4,
2. Consolidate flows at HSA level, shown in Figure 4.5,

---

[1] For more details on how to create or clone an environment in ArcGIS Pro, visit: https://pro.arcgis.com/en/pro-app/latest/arcpy/get-started/work-with-python-environments.htm.

[2] The tool "Generate Spatial Weights Matrix" in the current ArcGIS Pro 2.7 generates a ".swm" file, and the tool of converting it to a table does not work on some computers.

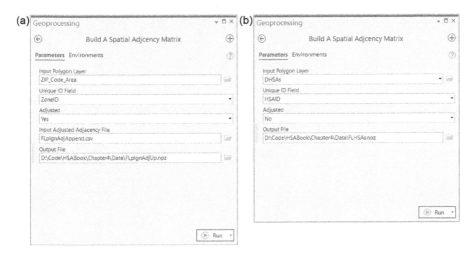

FIGURE 4.4
Interface for building a spatial adjacency matrix from (a) ZIP codes and (b) HSAs.

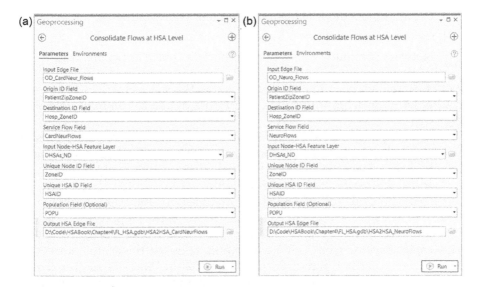

FIGURE 4.5
Interface for consolidating (a) cardiovascular surgery and neurosurgery flows at the ZIP code level to HSA level and (b) neurosurgery flows at ZIP code level to HSA level.

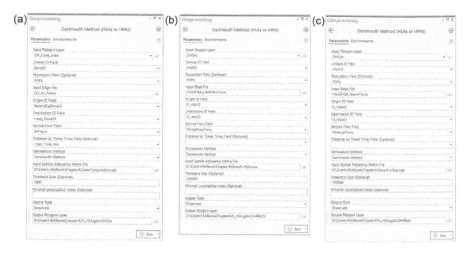

FIGURE 4.6
Interface of the refined Dartmouth method in defining (a) HSAs from hospitalization flows,
(b) HRRs from cardiovascular surgery and neurosurgery combined flows, and (c) HRRs from
neurosurgery flows.

3. Dartmouth method (HSAs or HRRs), shown in Figure 4.6,

4. Calculate regionalization indices, shown in Figure 4.7, and

5. Network community detection method (ScLeiden or ScLouvain).

Tools 1–4 are illustrated in more detail below. The last tool will be discussed
in Chapter 6 for delineating HSAs and HRRs by the community detection
approach.

Before using these tools, ensure that the Script File of each tool points to
the same Python script under the folder `Scripts`. Specially, right-click each
tool and select Properties to open the dialog window of Tool Properties. In
the General tab, verify the path of Script File.

The first tool "`Build A Spatial Adjacency Matrix`", as shown in
Figure 4.4, constructs a spatial adjacency matrix between polygons, such as
ZIP code areas or HSAs. The Input Polygon Layer must have a Unique ID Field
with values starting from 1. If a user wants to adjust the spatial adjacency
matrix when some polygons are separated by natural barriers, such as rivers,
lakes, or mountains, but are bridged by some man-made infrastructure, select
"`Yes`" for Adjusted and a csv file for the Input Adjusted Adjacency File (as
shown in Figure 4.4a). Otherwise, leave the default setting "`No`" for Adjusted
(as shown in Figure 4.4b). For example, for two polygons with `ZoneID=3` and
`ZoneID=4` that are not spatially adjacent but are connected by a bridge, the
adjusted adjacency file (e.g., `FLplgnAdjAppend.csv`) contains one row with
two column values such as "3, 4", which correspond to origin `ZoneID` and
destination `ZoneID`. Note that there is no header name for the two columns.
The Output File name ends with ".npz", a file format to store array data by the

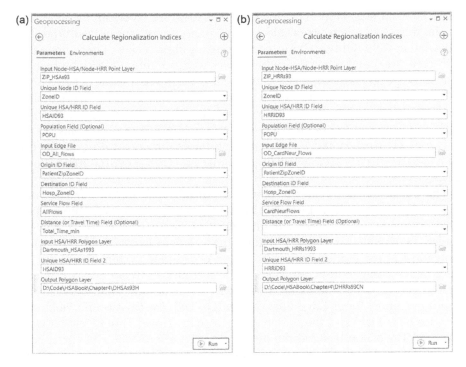

FIGURE 4.7
Interface of calculating regionalization indices for (a) 1993 Dartmouth HSAs and (b) 1993 Dartmouth HRRs.

NumPy package. The .npz file format can improve computational efficiency when using a large spatial adjacency matrix to delineate HSAs or HRRs. This tool also outputs the same spatial adjacency matrix in a csv file format under the same path. The csv file only includes polygons that are spatially adjacent and has three columns representing origin ID field, destination ID field, and weight (=1). Users can join the geographic coordinates of origin ID field and destination ID field and then use the "XY To Line" tool in ArcGIS Pro to generate a flow map and validate whether the adjacent polygons are linked by lines or not. Appendix B provides a detailed illustration about the usage of this tool.

The second tool "Consolidate Flows at HSA Level", as shown in Figure 4.5, is designed to consolidate flows between areas at a finer level (i.e., ZIP codes, census tracts, or census blocks) to flows between areas at a coarser level (e.g., flows between HSAs needed for defining HRRs). The Input Edge File must be a table in geodatabase, with (1) a unique Origin ID Field and (2) a unique Destination ID Field with both values starting from 1, and (3) a Service Flow Field between the two (e.g., flow from an origin ZIP code area to a destination ZIP code area). The Input Node-HSA Feature Layer must have two fields, a Unique Node ID Field (e.g., ZIP code area ID) and a Unique

HSA ID Field (e.g., HSA ID). This node-HSA feature layer can be generated in the third tool when users select "Not dissolved" for output type. The Population Field (Optional) represents the population size of each node (i.e., ZIP code area) and is needed when users want to define HRRs by using a threshold population size. The Output HSA Edge File for the service flows between HSAs is saved in a table. As mentioned above, this tool is mainly used to prepare HSA-to-HSA flows from the ZIP-to-ZIP flows for defining HRRs. If users are only interested in defining HSAs, there is no need to use this tool. Figure 4.5a and b shows the interfaces for aggregating (a) the cardiovascular surgery and neurosurgery flows and (b) the neurosurgery flows, respectively.

The third tool "Dartmouth Method (HSAs or HRRs)", as shown in Figure 4.6, defines HSAs or HRRs by the refined Dartmouth method. There are three items associated with the input polygon feature: Input Polygon Layer, its Unique ID Field, and the optional Population Field. The input polygon feature should have a projected coordinate system to ensure the geographic compactness, an index to be introduced in Section 4.4, is calibrated properly. Five items are associated with the flow data between the input polygons: Input Edge File, Origin ID Field, Destination ID Field, and Service Flow Field and the optional Distance (or Travel Time) Field between the two. The origin IDs and the destination IDs are unique and correspond to the unique IDs in the input polygon layer. Two Delineation Methods are provided, Dartmouth Method and Huff–Dartmouth Method. The former option relies on actual flows, and the latter option uses estimated flows from the Huff model (to be discussed in Chapter 5). The Input Spatial Adjacency Matrix File is generated by the first tool, Build A Spatial Adjacency Matrix, and its rows and columns correspond to the values of the unique ID fields−1 in the input polygon layer. The Threshold Size and Minimum Localization Index are designed for users to impose rule (1) and/or rule (2) in the refined Dartmouth method (discussed in Sub-section 4.2.1).

For defining HSAs, the default values of 1,000 and 0.5 are set for threshold size and LI, respectively. Note that the usage of threshold size requires a population field with non-zero population for polygon features. Various choices for these two items lead to four scenarios:

1. HSAs without any constraints of threshold size or minimum LI,
2. HSAs with a threshold size only,
3. HSAs with a minimum LI only, and
4. HSAs with both the constraints of threshold size and minimum LI.

For defining HRRs, users can change the default values to 120,000 and 0.65 for threshold size and LI, respectively.

The Output Type has two options, "Dissolved" and "Not dissolved". The option "Dissolved" is used to define contiguous HSAs (or HRRs) and calculates several regionalization indices in the newly derived HSAs (or HRRs). These indices (e.g., LI, compactness) will be discussed in Section 4.4. Users may choose the option "Not dissolved" to prepare a node-HSA feature layer used in the second tool to consolidate ZIP-to-ZIP flows to HSA-to-HSA flows for defining HRRs. In other words, it prepares a layer identical to the input polygon layer with an additional field to identify which ZIP code areas (finer-level area unit) are contained in which HSAs (coarser-level area unit), or which HSAs are contained in which HRRs. Figure 4.6a–c shows the interfaces for defining (a) HSAs from all hospitalization flows between ZIP code areas, (b) HRRs from cardiovascular surgery and neurosurgery combined flows between HSAs, and (c) HRRs from neurosurgery flows between HSAs, respectively. If users already have the HSA polygon layer and a table of flows between HSAs and want to define HRRs using this tool, ensure that the HSA layer has a unique HSAID field to identify each HSA. Also, if users want to compute the number of hospitals within each HRR, ensure that there is a Num _ DZoneID field with values in Integer type that corresponds to the destination HSAID field in the same flow table.

The fourth tool "Calculate Regionalization Indices", as shown in Figure 4.7, uses the flow data to calculate some common indices for assessing regionalization outcomes. There are four items associated with the input point layer: the Input Node-HSA/Node-HRR Point Layer that contains the relationship of the ZIP code areas vs. HSAs (or HSAs vs. HRRs), its Unique Node ID Field, Unique HSA/HRR ID Field, and the optional Population Field of each node. Note that this input layer can be a result of the third tool when the option of "Not dissolved" is chosen or a point layer prepared by users to specify the relationship between ZIP code and HSAs. There are five items associated with the flow data between the nodes: Input Edge File, its Origin ID Field, Destination ID Field, and the Service Flow Field and optional Distance (or Travel Time) Field between the two. The unique origin ID field and unique destination ID field correspond to the unique node ID field in the input point layer. It suggests that the flow data should be consolidated at the same level as the input point layer. Moreover, two items are associated with the dissolved HSAs (HRRs): Input HSA/HRR Polygon Layer and its Unique HSA/HRR ID Field 2, which are used to join the newly calibrated indices and generate the output polygon layer. The result has identical features to the input HSA/HRR polygon layer but with more attributes, such as the number of nodes, the number of destination nodes, LI, geographic compactness, population size, and average travel time, if the population field and distance field are chosen. Note that this tool is mainly designed for calculating regionalization indices for pre-existing areas, such as the 1993 Dartmouth HSAs (HRRs), in Sub-section 4.4.2. The newly derived HSAs and HRRs in the third tool already have these indices calculated. Figure 4.7a and b shows the interfaces for calculating regionalization indices for (a) 1993 Dartmouth HSAs and (b) 1993 HRRs, respectively.

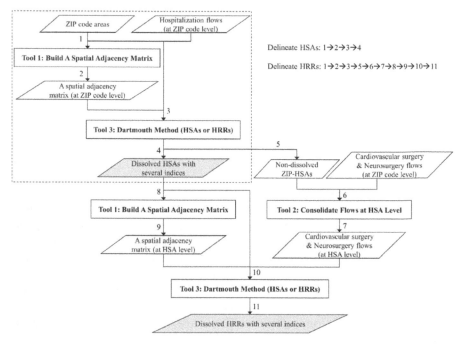

FIGURE 4.8
Workflow of using the three tools to delineate HSAs and HRRs by the refined Dartmouth method.

Figure 4.8 illustrates the workflow of using the four tools. In summary, the automated delineation of HSAs by the refined Dartmouth method (1) uses the first tool to build a spatial adjacency matrix between ZIP code areas and then (2) uses the third tool to define HSAs. After the HSAs are ready, the automated delineation of HRRs by the refined Dartmouth method (1) uses the third tool to construct a ZIP–HSA feature layer with the option "Not dissolved" in the output type, (2) uses the second tool to aggregate the ZIP-to-ZIP flows to the HSA-to-HSA flows, (3) uses the first tool to build a spatial adjacency matrix between HSAs, and (4) finally runs the third tool again (this time with the option "Dissolved" in the output type) to delineate HRRs from HSAs. Note that the third tool is used twice in defining HRRs: The first time is to replicate the process of delineating HSAs but with the option "Not dissolved" to preserve the ZIP–HSA containment relationship in order to facilitate the flow consolidation between HSAs (the second tool), and the second time is to construct HRRs from HSAs. The fourth tool is not needed either for defining HSAs or for defining HRRs, and it is only designed for the convenience of calibrating some regionalization indices for any area unit (in our case, the 1993 Dartmouth HSAs or HRRs for comparison discussed in Sub-section 4.4.2). The next Section 4.4 uses a case study to illustrate how to use these tools to delineate HSAs and HRRs in Florida.

4.4 Delineating HSAs and HRRs in Florida by the Refined Dartmouth Method

This case study uses the feature class ZIP _ Code _ Area and three tables OD _ All _ Flows, OD _ CardNeur _ Flows, and OD _ Neuro _ Flows under the geodatabase FL _ HSA.gdb to delineate HSAs and HRRs in Florida by the refined Dartmouth method. As introduced in Chapter 1, the feature class ZIP _ Code _ Area includes 983 ZIP code areas in Florida with field POPU for population in 2010, and the three tables include (1) 37,180 non-zero flows and 2,392,066 total service volumes for hospitalization, (2) 14,168 non-zero flows and 293,050 total service volumes for cardiovascular surgery and neurosurgery, and (3) 7,049 non-zero flows and 40,002 total service volumes for neurosurgery.

Figure 4.9a–c shows their spatial distributions of the major flows in terms of their percentages of total service volumes accordingly. See Appendix B for a user guide on how to use ArcGIS Pro to create these straight-line network flow maps.

4.4.1 Delineating HSAs and HRRs in Florida by the Automated Toolkit

The following process illustrates how to use the toolkit of "HSA Delineation Pro.tbx" to delineate HSAs in Florida by the refined Dartmouth method.

1. Use the tool "Build A Spatial Adjacency Matrix".
   As shown in Figure 4.4a, select the feature class ZIP _ Code _ Area for Input Polygon Layer and its ZoneID for Unique ID field, select Yes for Adjusted and FLplgnAdjAppend.csv under the same folder of FL _ HSA.gdb for Input Adjusted Adjacency File, select the path and set the file name with ".npz" format for Output File. Click Run to generate the spatial adjacency matrix named "FLplgnAdjUp. npz".

2. Use the tool "Dartmouth Method (HSAs or HRRs)".
   As shown in Figure 4.6a, select the feature class ZIP _ Code _ Area for Input Polygon Layer, its ZoneID for Unique ID Field, and POPU for Population Field. Select the table OD _ All _ Flows for Input Edge File, its PatientZipZoneID for Origin ID Field, its Hosp _ ZoneID for Destination ID Field, its AllFlows for Service Flow Field, and its Total _ Time _ min for Distance (or Travel Time) Field. Select Dartmouth Method for Delineation Method and FLplgnAdjUp.npz for Input Spatial Adjacency Matrix File.[3] Leave Threshold Size as the default value of 1,000 and Minimum

---

[3] If the .npz file cannot be loaded, users need to copy the full path of the spatial adjacency matrix (e.g., D:\Code\HSABook\Chapter4\Data\FLplgnAdjUp.npz).

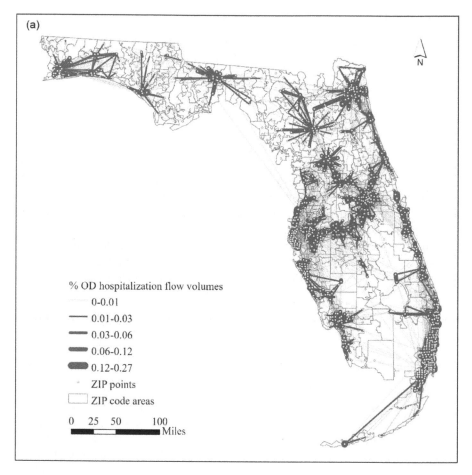

FIGURE 4.9

(a) Major flows (>=20) for all hospitalizations between ZIP code areas. (b) Major flows (>=5) for cardiovascular and neurosurgery patients between ZIP code areas. (c) Major flows (>=5) for neurosurgery patients between ZIP code areas.

(Continued)

Localization Index as blank. Select "Dissolved" for Output Type, and save the result as DHSAs. Click Run.

The feature class DHSAs has 136 spatially continuous HSAs. Open its attribute table. It has a field HSAID to identify each HSA, two fields COUNT _ ZoneID and Num _ DZoneID to record the number of ZIP code areas and the number of destination ZIP code areas (with hospitals) within each HSA, and four additional fields LI, POPU, Compactness, and EstTime to represent the LI, population size, geographic compactness, and average travel time of each HSA. The next Sub-section 4.4.2 will explain the definitions of these indices. If users want to generate HSAs with LI ≥0.5, input 0.5 for

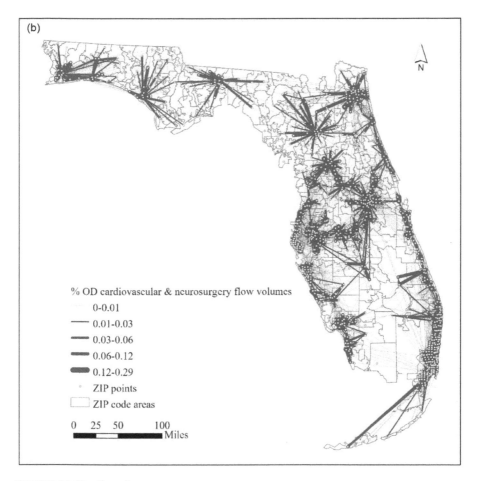

FIGURE 4.9 (*Continued*)
(a) Major flows (>=20) for all hospitalizations between ZIP code areas. (b) Major flows (>=5) for cardiovascular and neurosurgery patients between ZIP code areas. (c) Major flows (>=5) for neurosurgery patients between ZIP code areas.

(*Continued*)

Minimum Localization Index, change the name of the output polygon layer, and leave others as the above settings. Click Run again to generate a new set of HSAs.

The automated delineation of HRRs is similar, but has two more steps as the cardiovascular surgery and neurosurgery flows are provided at the ZIP code level. The following steps describe how to use the same toolkit to define HRRs in Florida by the refined Dartmouth method.

1. Use the tool "Dartmouth Method (HSAs or HRRs)".
    Use the same settings for all parameters as in Figure 4.6a, except for changing the Output Type to "Not dissolved" and naming

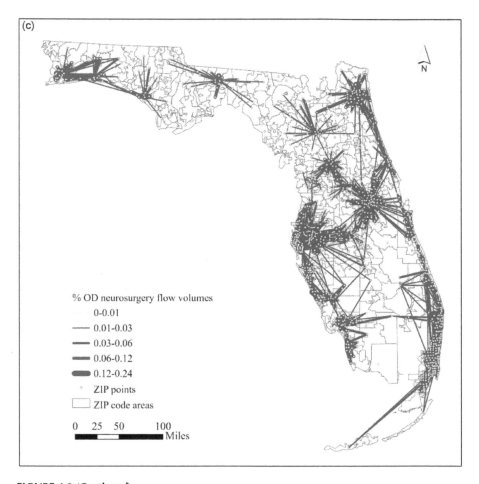

FIGURE 4.9 (Continued)
(a) Major flows (>=20) for all hospitalizations between ZIP code areas. (b) Major flows (>=5) for cardiovascular and neurosurgery patients between ZIP code areas. (c) Major flows (>=5) for neurosurgery patients between ZIP code areas.

the Output Polygon Layer to "DHSAs _ ND". Click Run to generate a ZIP–HSA polygon layer.

2. Use the tool "Consolidate Flows at HSA Level".

As shown in Figure 4.5a, select the table OD _ CardNeur _ Flows for Input Edge File, its PatientZipZoneID for Origin ID Field, Hosp _ ZoneID for Destination ID Field, and CardNeurFlows for Service Flow Field. Select the pre-defined non-dissolved feature class DHSAs _ ND for Input Node-HSA Feature Layer, and its ZoneID for Unique Node ID Field, HSAID for Unique HSA ID Field, and POPU for Population Field. Name the Output HSA Edge File as a table HSA2HSA _ CardNeurFlows. Click Run to consolidate the cardiovascular surgery and neurosurgery flows between ZIP codes areas to flows between HSAs.

The new table has 4,180 records with a total volume of 293,050, which is identical to the total service volume from the table OD _ CardNeur _ Flows. Open the attribute table. It has four important fields O _ HSAID, D _ HSAID, NCardNeurFlows, and Num _ DZoneID to represent the origin HSAID, destination HSAID, total service volumes between the two, and the number of destination ZIP codes within the destination HSA. Ensure that the name of the field Num _ DZoneID remains unchanged, and it will be used to calculate the total number of destination ZIP codes within each HRR.

3. Use the tool "Build A Spatial Adjacency Matrix".

As shown in Figure 4.4b, select the previously dissolved HSAs feature class DHSAs for Input Polygon Layer, choose its HSAID for Unique ID Field, leave Adjusted as default value "No", and name the Output File as FLHSAs.npz. Click Run to generate a spatial adjacency matrix between HSAs.

4. Use the tool "Dartmouth Method (HSAs or HRRs)" again.

As shown in Figure 4.6b, select the previously dissolved HSAs feature class DHSAs for Input Polygon Layer, and choose its HSAID for Unique ID Field and POPU for Population Field. Select the consolidated flows HSA2HSA _ CardNeurFlows from step 2 for Input Edge File, O _ HSAID for Origin ID Field, D _ HSAID for Destination ID Field, and NCardNeurFlows for Service Flow Field. Leave the Distance (or Travel Time) Field blank. Select Dartmouth Method for Delineation Method. Select FLHSAs.npz from step 3 for Input Spatial Adjacency Matrix File. Input 120,000 for Threshold Size, and leave the Minimum Localization Index blank. Choose Dissolved for Output Type, and name the Output Polygon Layer as DHRRsCN. Click Run.

The result is automatically loaded in the Contents pane. The feature class DHRRsCN has 59 spatially continuous HRRs, and each HRR has a population size greater than 120,000. Open the attribute table. It has a field HRRID to identify each HRR, three fields COUNT _ HSAID, Num _ DHSAID, and Num _ DZoneID to record the number of HSAs, the number of destination HSAs, and the number of destination ZIP codes within each HRR, and three additional fields LI, POPU, and Compactness to represent the LI, population size, and geographic compactness of each HRR. If users want to generate HRRs with LI ≥0.65, input 0.65 for Minimum Localization Index, change the name of the output polygon layer, and leave others as the above settings. Click Run to generate a new set of HRRs.

As stated in Sub-section 4.2.2, there is a need to reconsider the use of the combined cardiac and neurosurgery in defining the HRRs. Here, we explore the use of neurosurgery alone as the specialized hospital care for defining

HRRs. The process is similar. Steps 1 and 3 are the same, and the following outlines only steps 2 and 4 that are different.

In step 2, double-click the tool "Consolidate Flows at HSA Level" to open the dialog window. As shown in Figure 4.5b, select the table OD _ Neuro _ Flows for Input Edge File, PatientZipZoneID for Origin ID Field, Hosp _ ZoneID for Destination ID Field, and NeuroFlows for Service Flow Field. Select the pre-defined non-dissolved feature class DHSAs _ ND for Input Node-HSA Feature Layer, ZoneID for Unique Node ID Field, HSAID for Unique HSA ID Field, and POPU for Population Field. Name the Output HSA Edge File as a table HSA2HSA _ NeuroFlows. Click Run to consolidate the neurosurgery flows between ZIP codes areas to flows between HSAs. It also has four important fields O _ HSAID, D _ HSAID, NNeuroFlows, and Num _ DZoneID to represent the origin HSAID, destination HSAID, total service volumes between HSAs, and the number of destination ZIP codes within the destination HSA.

In step 4, double-click the tool "Dartmouth Method (HSAs or HRRs)" to open the dialog window. As shown in Figure 4.6c, select the previously dissolved HSAs feature class DHSAs for Input Polygon Layer, its HSAID for Unique ID Field, and its POPU for Population Field. Select the consolidated flows HSA2HSA _ NeuroFlows from step 2 for Input Edge File, O _ HSAID for Origin ID Field, D _ HSAID for Destination ID Field, and NNeuroFlows for Service Flow Field. Leave the Distance (or Travel Time) Field blank. Select Dartmouth Method for Delineation Method. Select FLHSAs.npz from step 3 for Input Spatial Adjacency Matrix File. Input 120,000 for Threshold Size, and leave the Minimum Localization Index blank. Choose Dissolved for Output Type, and save the HRRs feature class as DHRRsN under the geodatabase FL _ HSA.gdb. Click Run.

The result is automatically loaded in the Contents pane. Similarly, if users want to generate HRRs with the LI ≥0.65, input 0.65 for Minimum Localization Index, change the name of the output polygon layer, and leave others as the above settings. Click Run again to generate a new set of HRRs.

As illustrated in Figure 4.10, using a population threshold size of 1,000 for HSAs, the refined Dartmouth method generates 136 HSAs. Using a population threshold size of 120,000 for HRRs, those 136 HSAs are then aggregated to 59 HRRs based on the combined cardiovascular surgery and neurosurgery flows, or 48 HRRs based on the neurosurgery flows alone. By imposing the additional LI constraints of 0.5 and 0.65 for HSAs and HRRs, respectively, the refined Dartmouth method aggregates 136 HSAs to 74 HSAs, 35 HRRs based on the combined cardiovascular surgery and neurosurgery flows, and 18 HRRs based on the neurosurgery alone. The results are reported in Tables 4.1–4.3.

4.4.2 Calculating Indices for 1993 Dartmouth HSAs and HRRs in Florida by the Toolkit

The Dartmouth HSAs and HRRs defined in 1993 are downloaded from the Dartmouth Atlas of Health Care Project (https://www.dartmouthatlas.

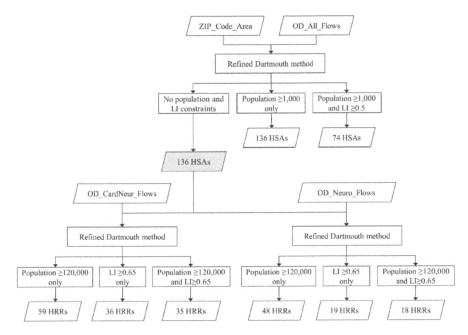

FIGURE 4.10
Workflow to delineating HSAs and HRRs with different constraints.

org/downloads/geography/). After overlapping those with the boundary of ZIP _ Code _ Area, we have extracted two feature classes Dartmouth _ HSAs1993 and Dartmouth _ HRRs1993 with 117 HSAs and 19 HRRs in Florida, respectively, and saved them under the geodatabase FL _ HSA.gdb. Some of the HSAs and HRRs across the state borders are thus clipped to contain only the parts in Florida. Data needed for calculating the indices also include the feature class ZIP _ Points and three tables OD _ All _ Flows, OD _ CardNeur _ Flows, and OD _ Neuro _ Flows under the same geodatabase.

The indices include the number of ZIP code areas, the number of destination ZIP code areas, LI, geographic compactness, population size, and average travel time. The number of ZIP code areas refers to those generating hospitalization patients, or origin ZIP code areas. The number of destination ZIP code areas refers to ZIP code areas with at least one hospital. *Localization index (LI)* refers to the proportion of hospitalizations that are in the same region as where the patients live. This study defines LI as the ratio of service flows within a region (HSA or HRR) divided by the total service flows originated from the same region. *Geographic compactness* describes the regularity of a region's shape based on the corrected perimeter-to-area ratio or $PAC = P / \left(3.54\sqrt{A}\right)$, where P denotes perimeter and A denotes area. Population size is the total population in a region, an index used for measuring balance of region size. Average travel time is the weighted average travel time for patients originated from the same region and reflects the overall travel burden for patients.

The following illustrates how these indices are calculated by using the automated toolkit. Step 1 is prepared for users who are interested in applying the tool for other study areas and can be skipped.

1. Identify the ZIP codes within each HSA or HRR.

   Open the attribute table of the feature class `Dartmouth_HSAs1993`, add a field `HSAID93` in Long data type, and calculate its unique value equal to the field `HSA_BDRY_I`. Similarly, open the attribute table of the feature class `Dartmouth_HRRs1993`, add a field `HRRID93` also in Long data type, and calculate its unique value equal to the field `HRR_BDRY_I`.

   Under Analysis, click Tools to open the Geoprocessing pane, search for "Spatial Join" and click on it to activate the dialog window. Select `ZIP_Points` for Target Features and `Dartmouth_HSAs1993` for Join Features, and name the Output Feature Class as "`ZIP_HSAs93`". Select Join one to one for Join Operation and Within for Match Option. Leave others default and click Run. Do the same for the feature class `Dartmouth_HRRs1993`, and name the Output Feature Class as "`ZIP_HRRs93`".

   Open the attribute tables of two feature classes `ZIP_HSAs93` and `ZIP_HRRs93`, check the features with null values of fields `HSAID93` and `HRRID93`, respectively, and fill the values if the ZIP code areas overlap the Dartmouth HSAs or HRRs. These two feature classes have already been prepared under the geodatabase `FL_HSA.gdb`. This step is illustrated for those who want to replicate the work on a different study area.

2. Calculate indices for 1993 Dartmouth HSAs.

   Activate the tool "`Calculate regionalization indices`" under the toolkit "`HSA Delineation Pro.tbx`". As shown in Figure 4.7a, select `ZIP_HSAs93` for Input Node-HSA/Node-HRR Point Layer, `ZoneID` for Unique Node ID Field, `HSAID93` for Unique HSA/HRR ID Field, and `POPU` for Population Field. Select `OD_All_Flows` for Input Edge File, `PatientZipZoneID` for Origin ID Field, `Hosp_ZoneID` for Destination ID Field, `AllFlows` for Service Flow Field, and `Total_Time_min` for Distance (or Travel Time) Field. Select `Dartmouth_HSAs1993` for Input HSA/HRR Polygon Layer and `HSAID93` for Unique HSA/HRR ID Field 2. Name Output Polygon Layer as "`DHSAs93H`", and click Run to calculate indices for each HSA.

3. Calculate indices for 1993 Dartmouth HRRs.

Like step 2, activate the same tool. As shown in Figure 4.7b, select ZIP _ HRRs93 for Input Node-HSA/Node-HRR Point Layer, its ZoneID for Unique Node ID Field, its HRRID93 for Unique HSA/ HRR ID Field, and its POPU for Population Field. Select OD _ CardNeur _ Flows for Input Edge File, its PatientZipZoneID for Origin ID Field, Hosp _ ZoneID for Destination ID Field, and CardNeurFlows for Service Flow Field, and leave the Distance (or Travel Time) Field blank. Select Dartmouth _ HRRs1993 for Input HSA/HRR Polygon Layer and HRRID93 for Unique HSA/HRR ID Field 2. Name Output Polygon Layer as "DHRRs93CN", and click Run to calculate indices for each HRR.

Repeat the same step for the HRRs based on the neurosurgery flows alone. That is, select OD _ Neuro _ Flows for Input Edge File and NeuroFlows for Service Flow Field, name the Output Polygon Layer as "DHRRs93N", and leave others the same. Click Run.

The indices of 1993 Dartmouth HSAs based on all hospitalization flows and HRRs based on cardiovascular surgery and neurosurgery flows combined and neurosurgery flows alone are obtained and will be used as the baseline to compare with those delineated from the refined Dartmouth method in the next sub-section.

4.4.3 Evaluating HSAs and HRRs by the Refined Dartmouth Method

To evaluate the quality of HSAs and HRRs derived by the refined Dartmouth method, we select three common indices from health care studies for comparisons: LI, geographic compactness, and balanced region size. LI represents the tendency of patients to seek local hospitalization and is considered as the most important property in health care service area delineation. A higher LI is more favorable as it demonstrates that generated HSAs or HRRs better reflect local health care markets. Geographic compactness and balanced region size are two other measures widely used to assess the quality of regionalization from a geographic perspective (Guo, 2008). A lower PAC value implies a more compact region that is more acceptable in system planning. Balanced region size is often desirable so that regions are comparable in population size. Other indices such as the number of origin ZIP code areas, the number of destination ZIP code areas, and average travel time are only for information.

Table 4.1 shows the comparison of the two scenarios of our newly derived HSAs to the 117 original Dartmouth HSAs. The minimum population size of 1,000 is imposed to avoid extremely small HSAs and does not take effect in our case. The refined Dartmouth method generates 136 HSAs without imposing any minimum LI criterion, largely in line with the number (117) of original HSAs. With an enforcement of LI≥0.5, the refined Dartmouth method

TABLE 4.1

Indices for HSAs in Florida

Indices		HSAs by Refined Dartmouth Method		Original Dartmouth HSAs (1993)
		Population ≥1,000[a]	Population ≥1,000 and LI >= 0.5	No Constraints
No. of HSAs		136	74	117
No. of destination ZIP code areas	Total	208	208	208
	Mean	2	3	2
	Min	1	1	0[b]
	Max	7	13	14
	S.D.	1	3	2
Localization index (LI)	Mean	0.513	0.667	0.515
	Min	0.188	0.508	0
	Max	1	1	0.946
	S.D.	0.153	0.121	0.219
Population (in 1,000)	Mean	138	254	161
	Min	6	14	1
	Max	602	1,384	1,908
	S.D.	121	278	250
Geographic compactness (PAC)	Mean	2.200	2.362	2.402
	Min	1.267	1.413	1.143
	Max	7.258	6.873	11.154
	S.D.	0.771	0.924	1.600
Average travel time (minute)	Mean	21.734	21.198	26.065
	Min	5.325	5.325	8.591
	Max	91.996	65.111	91.062
	S.D.	12.776	9.779	15.901

Note: S.D. stands for standard deviation.
[a] The same HSAs are derived without this constraint.
[b] Five HSAs do not have any hospitals.

derives 74 HSAs. Understandably, the consolidated and larger 74 HSAs enjoy a much higher mean LI (0.667) than the 117 original HSAs (0.551). As HSAs are defined to capture the basic hospital care markets, a larger number of HSAs are also more desirable and indicate an improved resolution. Our discussion now focuses on the 136 newly derived HSAs in comparison with the 117 original Dartmouth HSAs. The moderate increase in the number of HSAs (19) reflects an expanded health care market with more hospitals over time. More importantly, each of the 136 HSAs derived by the refined Dartmouth method contains at least one hospital, while five of the 117 original Dartmouth HSAs have no hospitals inside. It demonstrates the change of health care market for about two decades. Moreover, the increase in the

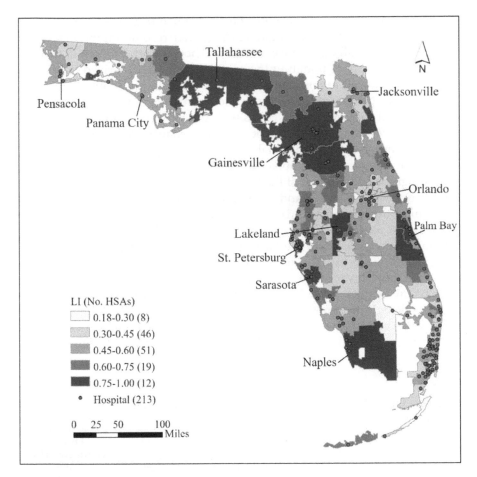

FIGURE 4.11
Localization index in 136 HSAs by the refined Dartmouth method.

HSA number comes with very little cost to the average LI value (0.513 vs. 0.515)[4] and more favorable (smaller) variability in standard deviation (0.153 vs. 0.219). Finally, the 136 HSAs have a lower standard deviation of population (121,000 vs. 250,000) and thus a more balanced region size, and also a smaller average PAC (2.2 vs. 2.402) and thus better geographic compactness. Figure 4.11 shows the variation of LI across 136 HSAs. The health care markets are more interwoven with lower LI values in cities such as Pensacola, Panama City, Jacksonville, and Orlando and are more localized with higher LI values in cities such as Tallahassee, Gainesville, Lakeland, St. Petersburg, Sarasota, Naples, and Palm Bay.

---

[4] In general, a larger number of HSAs and thus smaller HSAs on average imply that fewer hospitalization flows could be captured within HSAs and therefore lower LI values.

In summary, in comparison with the 1993 Dartmouth HSAs, the refined Dartmouth method generates more HSAs (better resolution) without much loss in LI, ensures all HSAs have at least one hospital, and therefore demonstrates the necessity of updating the original HSAs. The derived HSAs also enjoy more balanced region size and are more compact in shape.

Based on the cardiovascular surgery and neurosurgery flows, the 136 HSAs are aggregated to 59, 36, and 35 HRRs with different constraints of threshold population size and LI, and the results are reported in Table 4.2. All HRRs contain at least one specialized hospital, and Table 4.2 reports LI, population, and PAC for the assessment of regionalization quality. The impact of LI constraint is more significant than that of the threshold population size on reducing the number of HRRs (59 vs. 36), and the enforcement of both constraints only further reduces the number by 1 (i.e., to 35 HRRs). Given the purpose of HRRs for capturing the tertiary hospital markets, it is more realistic to believe that both constraints are enforced in the HRR delineation by the Dartmouth method. This yields 35 HRRs by the refined Dartmouth method, which are significantly more than, but closest to the 19 original HRRs in number of HRRs. Our discussion now focuses on the 35 newly derived HRRs in comparison with the 19 original HRRs. With almost twice as many HRRs, the new HRRs have an average LI value of 0.804, i.e., 4.5% decline from that of the original HRRs (0.842), but much less variability in LI (0.083 vs. 0.156 in standard deviation). The new

TABLE 4.2

Indices for HRRs Based on Cardiovascular Surgery and Neurosurgery Flows in Florida

Indices		HRRs by Refined Dartmouth Method			Original Dartmouth HRRs (1993)
		Population ≥120,000	LI≥0.65	Population ≥120,000 and LI≥0.65	Population ≥120,000 or LI≥0.65
No. of HRRs		59	36	35	19
Localization index (LI)	Mean	0.654	0.814	0.804	0.842
	Min	0.310	0.680	0.679	0.272
	Max	0.971	0.983	0.984	0.989
	S.D.	0.167	0.082	0.083	0.156
Population (in 1,000)	Mean	319	522	537	987
	Min	124	90	125	72
	Max	974	2,587	2,587	3,620
	S.D.	185	509	458	1,046
Geographic compactness (PAC)	Mean	2.399	2.566	2.610	3.359
	Min	1.308	1.425	1.425	1.580
	Max	5.526	5.526	5.526	5.705
	S.D.	0.933	1.071	1.077	1.230

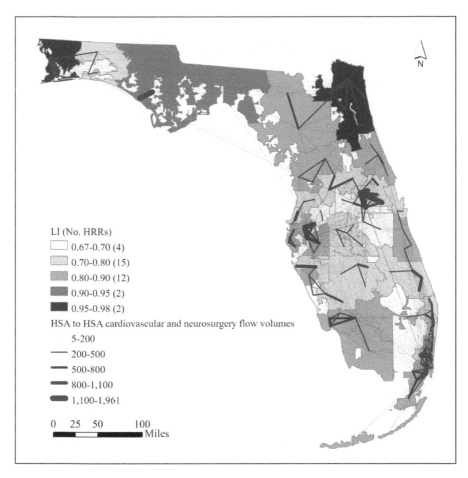

FIGURE 4.12
35 HRRs overlaid with major flows (≥5) for cardiovascular surgery and neurosurgery patients between HSAs.

HRRs are also more favorable in balanced region size (standard deviation of 458,000 vs. 1,046,000) and in compactness of shape (PAC mean value of 2.610 vs. 3.359). Figure 4.12 shows the 35 HRRs overlaid with major cardiovascular surgery and neurosurgery flows. Most major flows are enclosed in HRRs and demonstrate the value of plurality rule in the Dartmouth method.

As stated previously, this case study also explores the use of neurosurgery alone to define specialized hospital care and therefore examines the delineation of HRRs based on neurosurgery flows. The results are reported in Table 4.3. For similar reasoning, we focus on the scenario of 18 HRRs with both constraints on threshold population size and minimum LI, in comparison with the 19 original HRRs. With similar numbers of HRRs (18 vs. 19), the new HRRs now have a higher average LI value (0.822 vs. 0.745), a much

TABLE 4.3

Indices for HRRs Based on Neurosurgery Flows in Florida

Indices		HRRs by Refined Dartmouth Method			Original Dartmouth HRRs (1993)
		Population ≥120,000	LI≥0.65	Population ≥120,000 and LI≥0.65	Population ≥120,000 and LI≥0.65
No. of HRRs		48	19	18	19
Localization index (LI)	Mean	0.567	0.826	0.822	0.745
	Min	0.223	0.679	0.656	0.079
	Max	0.984	0.980	0.980	0.987
	S.D.	0.202	0.089	0.087	0.218
Population (in 1,000)	Mean	392	990	1,045	987
	Min	125	237	237	72
	Max	1,240	4,791	4,791	3,620
	S.D.	267	1,113	1,098	1,046
Geographic compactness (PAC)	Mean	2.513	3.163	3.321	3.359
	Min	1.314	1.746	1.850	1.579
	Max	6.523	6.524	6.524	5.705
	S.D.	1.073	1.252	1.196	1.230

narrow variability in LI (0.087 vs. 0.218 in standard deviation), a slightly more variability in region size (1,098,000 vs. 1,046,000 in standard deviation), and a slight edge in compactness of shape (PAC mean value of 3.321 vs. 3.359). Figure 4.13 shows the 18 HRRs overlaid with major neurosurgery flows.

One important finding from the case study is that the number of HRRs based on the cardiovascular surgery and neurosurgery flows, even when both constraints are enforced, remains high (35), almost double the number of original Dartmouth HRRs (19). Some recent literature argues that the increasing prevalence of cardiovascular surgery has made it less specialized (Hu et al., 2018). The number of HRRs based on the neurosurgery flows alone is 18, very close to the 19 original HRRs. Does this suggest that neurosurgery could be a better candidate to characterize specialized hospital care and be used for defining HRRs? What other medical services could be a better choice? This calls for more work from the public health professionals.

4.5 Summary

This chapter introduced the Dartmouth method for defining HSAs and HRRs. HSAs are constructed from ZIP code areas by using all hospitalization data

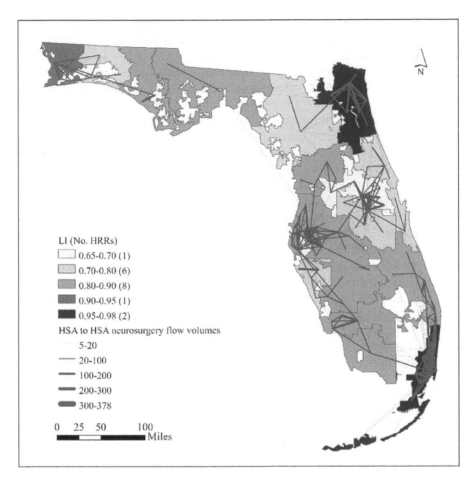

FIGURE 4.13
18 HRRs overlaid with major flows (≥5) for neurosurgery patients between HSAs.

in order to capture local hospital care market. HRRs are made of HSAs by using specialized care (e.g., cardiovascular surgery and neurosurgery) data in order to capture tertiary hospital care market. The Dartmouth method is the earliest attempt and remains the most popular method for delineating the two units, and both Dartmouth HSAs and HRRs have been widely used in public health studies.

Several reasons highlight the urgency of refining the method and updating its derived units: being outdated, relying on the Medicare data representing one demographic group (65+ year old), and lack of automation. The core of the Dartmouth method uses a plurality rule by assigning a ZIP code area to an HSA or HRR with the maximum flow of patients. There are at least four uncertainties in the traditional Dartmouth method, namely "the large city problem", "the non-independent HSA problem", "the maximum hospitalization problem", and "the spatial non-contiguity problem". All are addressed in the refined Dartmouth method illustrated in this chapter in order to define HSAs and HRRs consistently.

The automation of the method is implemented in ArcGIS Pro by three tools grouped under one toolkit: "Build a spatial adjacency matrix", "Consolidate flows at HSA level", and "Dartmouth method (HSAs or HRRs)". Various combinations of constraints such as threshold population size and minimum LI can be accommodated, as well as specification on spatial connections between areas separated by geographic barriers. The automated toolkit generates HSAs and HRRs consistent with the guidance established by the Dartmouth Atlas of Health Care Project.

The case study in Florida (based on the 2011 SID data from the HCUP) illustrates the usage of the tools. While there were 117 HSAs and 19 HRRs in Florida in 1993 by the original Dartmouth method, our refined method yields 136 HSAs, 35 HRRs based on cardiovascular surgery and neurosurgery data, and 18 HRRs based on neurosurgery-only data. In comparison with the 1993 original units, the newly derived HSAs have a better resolution (more HSAs) with little loss in LI, with at least one hospital in each HSA, and are more balanced in region size and more compact in shape, and the new HRRs possess similar advantages. Both support the need of timely update of the HSA and HRR delineations, and automated delineations introduced in this chapter have made such an endeavor feasible and cost-efficient.

5

Delineating Hospital Service Areas by the Huff Model

As stated in Chapter 1, hospital service area (HSA) is a functional region. Much of the early application of functional region has been in trade area analysis, a common and important task in the site selection of a retail store. A *trade area* is "the geographic area from which the store draws most of its customers and within which market penetration is highest" (Ghosh and McLafferty, 1987, p.62). Defining trade areas for the existing or proposed stores helps project market potentials, determines the focus areas for promotional activities, and highlights geographic weakness in its customer base and others. The proximal area method and the Huff model are two popular approaches widely used in retail and marketing analysis. This chapter discusses how both the methods are adapted for delineating HSAs. The proximal area method simply assumes that patients only choose the nearest hospital for services, and thus an HSA is composed of areas sharing the same nearest hospital. In addition to the distance decay effect, the Huff model also considers that a more attractive hospital (e.g., larger and of higher quality) may outdraw a competitor that is closer to patients. Understanding the proximal area method helps us build the foundation for the Huff model, the focus of this chapter.

In comparison with the Dartmouth method discussed in Chapter 4, the proximal area method or the Huff model has much less data need. Implementing the proximal area method only needs data of locations of hospitals and patients, and for the Huff model, additional measures such as hospital size and distance decay coefficient are also needed. The Dartmouth method utilizes the actual patient service flow data between residences of patients and hospitals in order to assign areas to hospitals being visited most often, i.e., the plurality rule. In the absence of such actual origin-destination (OD) service flow data, the proximal area method or the Huff model may be considered. In fact, the core of the Huff model is to estimate or predict such OD flows. In addition to data availability, another issue that necessitates the use of Huff model is the need to evaluate the impact of various planning scenarios such as hospital closures or openings on market reconfiguration.

Section 5.1 discusses the proximal area method and its GIS implementation in a case study. The case study demonstrates two approaches: One defines proximity by Euclidean distance and another by travel time through

DOI: 10.1201/9780429260285-5

a road network. The latter needs access to the Network Analysis module, introduced in Sub-section 2.2.2. Section 5.2 reviews the evolution of the Huff model over time and some refinement and extensions. The refinement uses a best-fitting distance decay function, discussed in Chapter 3, instead of being limited to a power function in the classic Huff model. Section 5.3 uses a case study to illustrate the step-by-step implementation of the Huff model in ArcGIS Pro. Section 5.4 introduces a toolkit that automates the Huff model's implementation, specifically the OD flow estimation part, and then uses the automated tool for refined Dartmouth method introduced in Section 4.3 for post-treatment to ensure spatial contiguity and other desirable properties for HSAs. As stated previously, all case studies in this chapter use the same data in Florida as detailed in Section 1.3. Section 5.5 concludes the chapter with a summary.

5.1 The Proximal Area Method and Its Implementation in GIS

A simple approach to defining HSAs is the *proximal area method*, which assumes that patients choose the nearest hospital among alternative facilities. The proximal area method implies that patients only consider distance (or travel time) in their choice of hospital cares, and thus a service area is simply made of residential areas of patients that are closer to the hospital than any other. How to define proximal areas in GIS depends on the measurement of spatial impedance. Here Sub-sections 5.1.1 and 5.1.2 illustrate how proximal areas are defined when spatial impedance is measured in Euclidean (or geodesic) distance and travel time, respectively.

5.1.1 Defining Proximal Areas in Euclidean Distance in GIS

When proximity is simply measured in Euclidean distance, we may define service areas by starting with either the hospital locations or the patients' residential locations. The former constructs Thiessen (or Voronoi) polygons from hospital locations, overlays the polygons with patient locations (e.g., a census tract or ZIP code area layer with population information) to identify patient areas within each polygon, and aggregates the data by the polygon IDs. For example, Roos (1993) used the Thiessen polygons to define HSAs. The latter utilizes a tool "Near" to identify the nearest hospital for each patient area and then integrates patient areas sharing identical hospital IDs to form the HSAs. The two are illustrated here and yield similar results, and the latter is recommended for its simplicity.

The *supply-based Thiessen approach* for defining proximal areas is implemented in the following three steps in ArcGIS Pro:

1. Generating the Thiessen polygons.

   Under Analysis, click Tools to open the Geoprocessing pane, search for "Create Thiessen Polygons" and click on it to activate the dialog window. Select Hosp_ZIP for Input Features, name the Output Feature Class as Hosp_ThiessenPoly, and accept the default setting "Only Feature ID" for Output Fields. Click Run. It generates 213 Thiessen polygons.

2. Identifying ZIP code areas whose population-weighted centroids fall within the Thiessen polygons.

   In the Contents pane, right-click the layer ZIP_Points>Joins and Relates>Spatial Join. Make sure that ZIP_Points is Target Features, select Hosp_ThiessenPoly for Join Features, name the Output Feature Class as ZIP_in_Thiessen, use "Join one to one" for Join Operation, check "Keep All Target Features", and select "Within" for Match Option. Click Run.

   Since ZIP_in_Thiessen is a point layer, join it to ZIP_Code_Area by the common field Zone_ID to transfer the field Input_FID to the polygon layer. Review the attribute table of ZIP_Code_Area, where the field Input_FID identifies the Thiessen polygons.

3. Defining the proximal areas.

   Under Analysis, click Tools to open the Geoprocessing pane, search for "Dissolve" and click on it to activate the dialog window. Select ZIP_Code_Area for Input Features, name the Output Feature Class as ProxArea_Thiessen, choose Input_FID for Dissolve Field, and POPU (Statistics Type "Sum") for Statistics Field(s). Click Run. It generates 212 proximal areas with population distribution as shown in Figure 5.1.

Note that one hospital (OBJECTID=210 on the feature Hosp_ZIP) is very close to several other hospitals and its Thiessen polygon is too small to contain any ZIP code area centroids, as shown in Figure 5.2a. In other words, no ZIP code areas identify it as their nearest hospital, and thus the total number of proximal areas (212) is one short of the total number of hospitals (213).

The *demand-based approach* for defining proximal areas is implemented in the following two steps in ArcGIS Pro:

1. Identifying the nearest hospitals from ZIP code areas.

   Under Analysis, click Tools to open the Geoprocessing pane, search for "Near" and click on it to activate the dialog window. Select ZIP_Points for Input Features and Hosp_ZIP for Near Features, and accept the default setting "Planar" for Method.[1] Click

---

[1] By choosing "Geodesic" for Method and completing the remaining process, one can generate proximal areas based on the geodesic distances. This option is more desirable for a large study area as discussed in Sub-section 2.2.1 in Chapter 2.

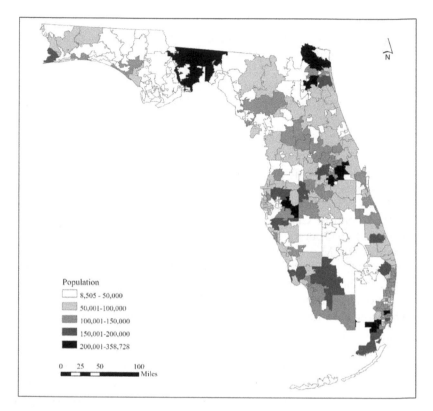

FIGURE 5.1
Hospital proximal areas based on Euclidean distances in Florida.

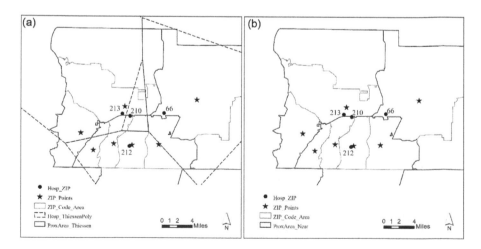

FIGURE 5.2
Illustration of problematic proximal areas: (a) by the hospitals-based Thiessen polygon approach; (b) by the Euclidean-distance-based nearest facility approach.

Run. The attribute table for the layer ZIP _ Points now has two new fields: NEAR _ FID identifies the nearest hospital from each ZIP code area (its population-weighted centroid), and NEAR _ DIST is the Euclidean distance between them in meters.[2]

Join ZIP _ Points to ZIP _ Code _ Area by the common field ZoneID to transfer two fields NEAR _ FID and NEAR _ DIST to the ZIP code areas in polygons.

2. Defining the proximity areas.

Under Analysis, click Tools to open the Geoprocessing pane, search for "Dissolve" and click on it to activate the dialog window. Select ZIP _ Code _ Area for Input Features, name the Output Feature Class as ProxArea _ Near, choose Near _ FID for Dissolve Field, and choose POPU (Statistics Type "Sum") for Statistics Field(s). Click Run. It generates 212 proximal areas.

Similar to the proximal areas defined by the hospitals-based Thiessen polygons, the same hospital (OBJECTID=210 on the feature Hosp _ ZIP) is not the nearest hospital for any ZIP code areas, as shown in Figure 5.2b.

The two methods derive the same HSAs, as shown in Figure 5.1. However, our experiments in other studies show that the two methods may yield largely consistent but slightly different service areas.

5.1.2 Defining Proximal Areas in Travel Time in GIS

When the spatial impedance is defined as the travel distance or time through a transportation network, we can use the tool "Closest Facility" in the ArcGIS Pro Network Analysis module to derive the proximal areas. The following steps implement the task.

1. Activating the Closest Facility tool.

In ArcGIS Pro, add related feature classes to the project (ZIP _ Code _ Area, ZIP _ Points, Hosp _ ZIP, FLRd2012). Under Analysis>Network Analysis, make sure that the network data source is FLRd _ ND, which is defined in Sub-section 2.2.2. Under Network Analysis, choose Closest Facility. A composite network analysis layer "Closest Facility" is added to the Contents pane.

2. Finding the nearest hospital for each ZIP code area.

Click the composite layer Closest Facility to select it. Click the Closest Facility tab under the Network Analysis group at the top

---

[2] One may also use a spatial join to accomplish the task. Specifically, right click ZIP _ Points > Joins and Relates > Spatial Join. Select ZIP _ Points as Target Features, select Hosp _ ZIP as Join Features, name Output Feature Class as ZIP _ Near _ Hosp, and select Closest as Match Option. Run.

of ArcGIS Pro to review the controls, including Import Facilities, Import Incidents, Travel Settings, and Run, to be defined as below[3]:

    a. Import Facilities: use `Hosp _ ZIP` to define Input Locations and use the default value 5,000 m to define Search Tolerance;

    b. Import Incidents: use `ZIP _ Points` to define Input Locations and use 10,000 m to define Search Tolerance;

    c. Travel Setting > Travel Mode: choose Driving for Type, and under Costs, define `Time _ min` for Impedance; and

    d. Click Run to execute the tool.
        The solution is saved in the layer `Routes`.

  3. Defining the proximal areas of hospitals.

      Join the attribute table of `Routes` to the layer `ZIP _ Points`,[4] whose `OBJECTID` is the same as the field `IncidentID` of `Routes`. Then join `ZIP _ Points` to `ZIP _ Code _ Area` by `ZoneID` to obtain the ZIP code areas in polygons.

      Under Analysis, click Tools and search for "Dissolve" and activate the tool. In the Dissolve tool dialog window, select `ZIP _ Code _ Area` for Input Features, name the Output Feature Class as `ProxArea _ Time`, choose `FacilityID` for Dissolve Field, and choose `POPU` for Statistics Field and "Sum" for corresponding Statistics Type. Click Run.

It generates 209 proximal areas with population distribution as shown in Figure 5.3. Four hospitals do not have their proximal areas, and thus the number of proximal areas is four short of the total number of hospitals (213).

Figure 5.4a–d illustrates the spatial locations of four hospitals with `OBJECTID`=32, 59, 90, and 213, respectively, on the feature layer `Hosp _ ZIP`. Boundary for each proximal area is in thick black, ZIP code points are in stars, the nearest hospitals are in circle dots, and the road paths are in dash lines. One common observation is that each of these four hospitals has another hospital nearby that is closer to the ZIP code area in its proximal area. For example, Figure 5.4a shows the hospital with `OBJECTID`=32 is very close to the one with `OBJECTID`=44, but the latter is the nearest and thus anchors the proximal area composed of the five ZIP code areas.

If a pre-defined OD travel time matrix is available, we can utilize the matrix to identify what patient areas share the same nearest hospitals and aggregate them by the hospital IDs accordingly. Recall that in Sub-section 2.2.2, an OD travel time table `OD _ All _ Flows` is calibrated by the "OD Cost

---

[3] If necessary, refer to Sub-section 2.2.2 on using the OD Cost Matrix tool, a similar process with more details.

[4] Do not join the table `Routes` to `ZIP _ Code _ Area` by the field name `OBJECTID` directly. Values for the field `OBJECTID` in `ZIP _ Code _ Area` are not identical to the values of `OBJECTID` in `ZIP _ Points`.

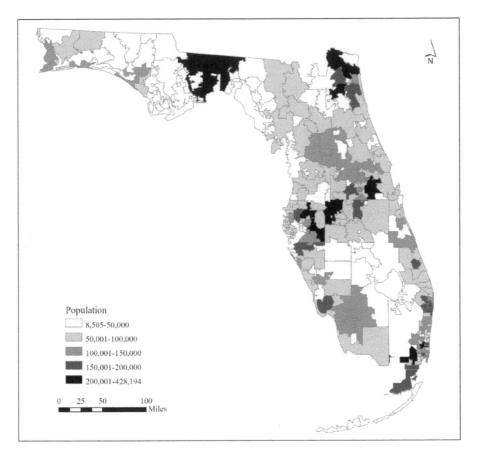

FIGURE 5.3
Hospital proximal areas based on travel time in Florida.

Matrix" tool in Network Analysis module, with fields: PatientZipZoneID for Origin ID Field, Hosp _ ZoneID for Destination ID Field, and Total _ Time _ min for Travel Time. The following outlines the process to construct the proximal areas for hospitals:

1. On the attribute table of OD _ All _ Flows, right-click the field PatientZipZoneID and select Summarize. OD _ All _ Flows becomes the Input Table; name the Output Table as HospMinTime; under Statistics Field(s), select Total _ Time _ min for Field and "Minimum" for its corresponding Statistic Type and make sure that the Case Field is PatientZipZoneID. Click Run.

2. Join the table HospMinTime back to OD _ All _ Flows based on the common field PatientZipZoneID. On the expanded table OD _ All _ Flows, select the records with the condition

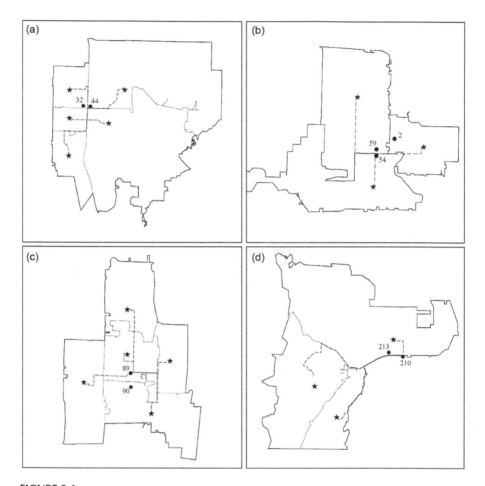

FIGURE 5.4
Travel-time-based proximal areas for hospitals with (a) OBJECTID=32, (b) OBJECTID=59, (c) OBJECTID=90, and (d) OBJECTID=213.

"MIN _ Total _ Time _ min = Total _ Time _ min" and export the result to a new table ProxTime.

3. Join the table ProxTime to the feature class ZIP _ Code _ Area by their corresponding common fields PatientZipZoneID and ZoneID, respectively.

4. Use Dissolve tool to aggregate ZIP _ Code _ Area by the field Hosp _ ZoneID, and choose POPU and NUMBEDS (Statistics Type "Sum" for both) for Statistics Field(s) to generate proximal areas.

To recap, the two methods based on Euclidean distance yield the same result with 212 proximal areas and the travel-time-based method derives 209 proximal areas. The difference is attributable to the specific distribution of hospitals, ZIP code centroids, and the road network connecting them. One nearest hospital from a ZIP code area in Euclidean distance may not remain the nearest via a road network. When several hospitals are near each other, some of them are not able to form their own proximal areas. In our case, it is more often the case for travel-time-based proximal areas than Euclidean-distance-based proximal areas. Conceivably, if the demand layer is in a higher resolution (i.e., a smaller analysis unit such as census block instead of ZIP code area), the number of hospitals without their own proximal areas is likely to be reduced or completely eliminated as the space is more divisible.

5.2 The Huff Model and Extensions

The proximal area method only considers distance or time in defining service areas. However, patients may bypass the closest hospital to patronize hospitals with higher-quality care, better reputation, more attractive price, or a larger selection of physicians. A hospital in proximity to other health care services (e.g., mental and physical therapies, rehabilitation) may also attract patients farther than an isolated hospital because of post-surgery recovery needs. The Huff model is based on the gravity model that considers two factors: distances (or time) from and attractions of hospitals. Sub-section 5.2.1 reviews the evolution of Huff model from Reilly's law and the relationship between them. Sub-section 5.2.2 introduces some extensions to the Huff model.

5.2.1 From Reilly's Law to the Huff Model

Reilly's law was developed for retail analysis (Reilly, 1931). Here it is discussed in the context of defining HSAs.

Consider two hospitals 1 and 2 that are at a distance of d_{12} from each other. Assume that the attractions for hospitals 1 and 2 are measured as S_1 and S_2 (e.g., in bed size), respectively. The question is to identify the *breaking point* (BP) that separates service areas of the two hospitals. The BP is d_{1x} from hospital 1 and d_{2x} from hospital 2, i.e.,

$$d_{1x} + d_{2x} = d_{12} \qquad (5.1)$$

By the notion of the *gravity model*, the gravitation by a hospital is proportional to its attraction and reversely related to the distance squared. Patients at the BP are indifferent in choosing either hospital, and thus the gravitations by the two hospitals are equal as follows:

$$S_1 / d_{1x}^2 = S_2 / d_{2x}^2 \qquad (5.2)$$

Using Equation 5.1, we obtain $d_{1x} = d_{12} - d_{2x}$. Substituting it into Equation 5.2 and solving for d_{1x} yield

$$d_{1x} = d_{12} / \left(1 + \sqrt{S_2 / S_1}\right) \tag{5.3}$$

Similarly,

$$d_{2x} = d_{12} / \left(1 + \sqrt{S_1 / S_2}\right) \tag{5.4}$$

Equations 5.3 and 5.4 define the boundary between the two HSAs, derived from Reilly's law.

The Reilly's law only defines service areas between two hospitals. A more general *Huff model* defines service areas of multiple hospitals (Huff, 1963). The model's widespread use and longevity "can be attributed to its comprehensibility, relative ease of use, and its applicability to a wide range of problems" (Huff, 2003, p.34).

Like in Equation 5.2, the gravitation of a hospital is positively related to the hospital's size, discounted by a distance decay effect (e.g., a power function) as $S_j d_{ij}^{-\beta}$. It is also referred to as *potential*, measuring the impact of a hospital j on a demand location i. The probability of a patient choosing a hospital j among a set of alternatives ($k=1, 2, ..., n$), P_{ij}, is equal to the proportion of that hospital's potential out of the total potentials of all hospitals such as

$$P_{ij} = S_j d_{ij}^{-\beta} / \sum_{k=1}^{n} \left(S_k d_{ik}^{-\beta}\right) \tag{5.5}$$

where S is the hospital's size, d is the distance, and $\beta > 0$ is the *distance friction coefficient*.

Equation 5.5 is the classic Huff model. Reilly's law may be considered as a special case of Huff model. In other words, when the distance friction coefficient β is assumed to be 2 and the choices are limited to two hospitals ($k=1, 2$), $P_{ij}=0.5$ defines the breaking point (BP) and the Huff model in Equation 5.5 is regressed to Reilly's law in Equation 5.2.

To illustrate the property of the Huff model, it is useful to stay with the simple Reilly's law, but assume a general friction coefficient β. Similar to Equation 5.2, we have

$$S_1 d_{1x}^{-\beta} = S_2 d_{2x}^{-\beta}$$

The BP is solved as

$$d_{1x} = d_{12} / \left[1 + (S_2 / S_1)^{1/\beta}\right], \text{ and}$$

$$d_{2x} = d_{12} / \left[1 + (S_1 / S_2)^{1/\beta}\right]$$

Therefore, if hospital 1 grows faster than hospital 2 (i.e., S_1 / S_2 increases), d_{1x} increases and d_{2x} decreases, indicating that the service area for hospital 1 expands at the cost of hospital 2. That is straightforward.

However, how does the change in β affect the service areas? When β decreases, if $S_1 > S_2$, i.e., $S_2 / S_1 < 1, (S_2 / S_1)^{1/\beta}$ decreases, and thus d_{1x} increases and d_{2x} decreases, indicating that a larger hospital is expanding its service area farther. That is to say, when the β value decreases over time due to improvements in transportation technologies or road network, travel impedance matters to a less degree, giving even a stronger edge to larger hospitals. This explains some of the challenges of small hospitals, especially those in rural areas, in the era of modern transportation and telecommunication technologies. According to the Sheps Center for Health Services Research (2021), 181 rural hospitals have closed since January 2005, and 138 closed since 2010, in the USA.

5.2.2 Extensions to the Huff Model

The original Huff model does not include an exponent associated with the facility (hospital) size. A simple improvement over the Huff model in Equation 5.5 is

$$P_{ij} = S_j^\alpha d_{ij}^{-\beta} / \sum_{k=1}^{n} \left(S_k^\alpha d_{ik}^{-\beta} \right)$$

where the exponent α captures elasticity of hospital size.

As discussed in Chapter 3, the distance decay effect may be best captured by a function different from the commonly used power function. The specific function and its associated parameter(s) should be derived from the actual travel data as in Sub-section 3.3.1. Using a general distance decay function $f(d)$, the refined Huff model is

$$P_{ij} = S_j f\left(d_{ij}\right) / \sum_{k=1}^{n} \left(S_k f\left(d_{ik}\right) \right) \tag{5.6}$$

where a unitary exponent for facility size S is adopted to preserve the model's simplicity and for other reasons discussed in Sub-section 3.3.1.

Another extension to the Huff model accounts for multiple factors associated with facilities such as history, reputation, accessibility, and other characteristics. Assuming these factors are multiplicative, the Huff model becomes a *multiplicative competitive interaction (MCI) model* (Nakanishi and Cooper, 1974) such as

$$P_{ij} = \left(\prod_{l=1}^{L} A_{lj}^{\alpha_l} \right) d_{ij}^{-\beta} / \sum_{k \in N_i} \left[\left(\prod_{l=1}^{L} A_{lk}^{\alpha_l} \right) d_{ik}^{-\beta} \right]$$

where A_{lj} is a measure of the lth ($l=1, 2, ..., L$) characteristic of hospital j, N_i is the set of hospitals considered by patients at i, and other notations are the same as in Equation 5.5.

For our case study, the empirical analysis from Sub-section 3.3.1 yields the power function as the best-fitting one with a friction coefficient of 1.43, which will be used in the next two sections on its GIS implementations.

5.3 Implementing the Huff Model for Delineating HSAs in ArcGIS Pro

Based on Equation 5.5, residents in an area visit hospitals with various probabilities, and an area is assigned to the service area of a hospital that is visited with the highest probability. If desirable, one may easily estimate the OD flows between residential areas and hospitals by multiplying the probabilities by demand size at each ZIP code area.

The following steps illustrate how to implement it in ArcGIS Pro. Figure 5.5 is the flow chart for the process. It begins with the OD flow table with the travel time attribute obtained from Sub-section 2.2.2.

1. Measuring hospital potentials
    Review the table OD _ All _ Flows, which contains fields from both the ZIP code areas (e.g., PatientZipZoneID, POPU) and

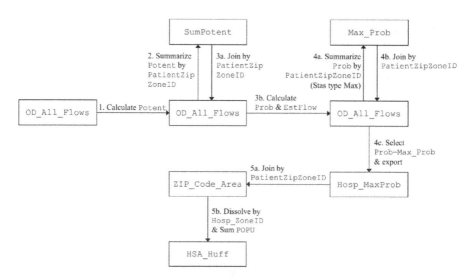

FIGURE 5.5
Workflow implementing the Huff Model in ArcGIS Pro.

the hospitals (e.g., Hosp _ ZoneID, NUMBEDS). Add a new field Potent (data type defined as Double), and calculate it as Potent =!NUMBEDS!*math.pow(!Total _ Time _ min!, -1.43) when the Expression Type is "Python 3" in default. The travel friction coefficient $\beta=1.43$ was derived in Sub-section 3.3.1.

This step computes the potential term $S_j d_{ij}^{-\beta}$ in Equation 5.5.

2. Calibrating total hospital potential for each ZIP code area

In contrast to the proximal area method that assigns a ZIP code area to the service area of its closest hospital, the Huff model considers the impact of hospital's attraction (here, its size in terms of number of beds) in addition to the distance (travel time) factor. A ZIP code area belongs to the service area of a hospital if the hospital (among 213 hospitals) is visited with the highest probability.

On the table OD _ All _ Flows, right-click the field PatientZipZoneID>Summarize. In the Summary Statistics dialog window, make sure that Input Table is OD _ All _ Flows and name Output Table as SumPotent; under Statistics Field(s), choose Potent for Field and "Sum" for corresponding Statistics Type, select PatientZipZoneID for Case field, and click Run. In the resulting table SumPotent, the field SUM _ Potent is the total potential for each ZIP code area.

This step computes the denominator $\sum_{k=1}^{n}\left(S_k d_{ik}^{-\beta}\right)$ in Equation 5.5. For each ZIP code area indexed by i, it has a unique value.

3. Calibrating the probability of each hospital being visited by each ZIP code area

   a. Join the table SumPotent back to OD _ All _ Flows (based on the common field PatientZipZoneID) to transfer the field SUM _ Potent.

   b. Add two new fields Prob and EstFlow (data type defined as Double for both) in OD _ All _ Flows, and calculate them as Prob=!Potent!/!SUM _ Potent!, and EstFlow =!Prob!*!POPU! when the Expression Type is "Python 3".

This step completes the calibration of probability $P_{ij} = S_j d_{ij}^{-\beta} / \sum_{k=1}^{n}\left(S_k d_{ik}^{-\beta}\right)$ in Equation 5.5, and multiplying it by the corresponding population in a ZIP code area yields the predicted patient flow from a ZIP code area i to a hospital j.

4. Identifying hospitals being visited with the highest probability

   a. On the table OD _ All _ Flows, right-click the field PatientZipZoneID, choose Summarize. In the Summary Statistics dialog window, make sure that Input Table is OD _ All _ Flows and name Output Table as MaxProb; under Statistics Field(s), choose Prob for Field and "Maximum" for corresponding Statistics Type, select `PatientZipZoneID` for Case field, and click Run. In the resulting table `MaxProb`, the field `MAX _ Prob` is the maximum probability for each ZIP code area to visit a particular hospital.

b. Join the table `MaxProb` back to `OD _ All _ Flows` (again, based on the common field `PatientZipZoneID`) to transfer the field `MAX _ Prob`.

c. Select records with the criterion `Prob` equal to `MAX _ Prob` (983 records selected). Right-click the Table `OD _ All _ Flows`, select Data and then Export Table to save the selected records to a table named `Hosp _ MaxProb`, which identifies the hospitals being visited by each ZIP code area with the highest probability.

If one replaces the field `Prob` by the field `EstFlow` and repeats this step, it yields the same result, i.e., identifying the same hospital experiencing the highest flow volume from a ZIP code area.[5]

5. Defining the HSAs by the Huff model

a. Join the table `Hosp _ MaxProb` to the feature class `ZIP _ Code _ Area` (recall that the values in field `PatientZipZoneID` of `Hosp _ MaxProb` correspond to those in field `ZoneID` of `ZIP _ Code _ Area`) to transfer two fields `MAX _ Prob` and `Hosp _ ZoneID`.

b. Similarly, use the tool "Dissolve" to aggregate `ZIP _ Code _ Area` by the field `Hosp _ ZoneID` and choose POPU and NUMBEDS (Statistics Type "Sum" for both) for Statistics Field(s) to derive the HSAs, named `HSA _ Huff`. Here, ZIP code areas visiting the same hospital with the highest probability are merged to form the HSA for that hospital.

The Huff model generates 166 HSAs as shown in Figure 5.6, where the values in parentheses represent the numbers of HSAs in corresponding ranges of population. Many small HSAs are distributed in the east and southwest coastal areas of Florida, while several larger HSAs are located in metropolitan areas, such as Tallahassee, Gainesville, Orlando, and Miami. As shown in Table 5.1, the population size varies from 3,662 in Valparaiso HSA to 2,076,116 in Miami HSA with a mean value of 113,272. The hospital size ranges from 15 beds in Live Oak HSA to 3,732 beds in Orlando HSA with a mean value of 366. Dividing the total number of hospital beds by population within each

---

[5] One may note the similarity between steps 2–3a and steps 4a–b. In fact, in step 2, in the Summary Statistics dialog, you may add another statistics field `Potent` with corresponding Statistics Type "Maximum", and then after step 3a, on the post-Join expanded table `OD _ All _ Flows`, select records with the criterion `Potent = MAX _ Potent`. It will identify the same hospital being visited most by each ZIP code area. This consolidates those steps by using the tools Summarize and Join once.

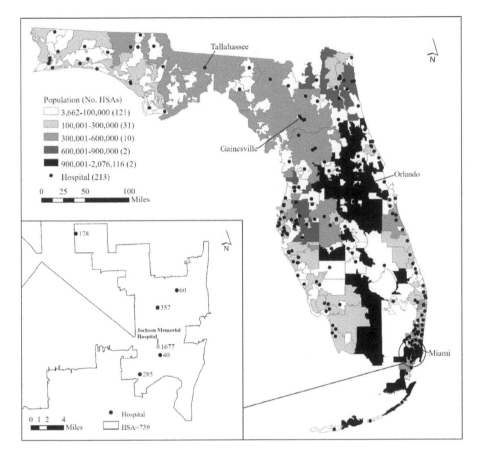

FIGURE 5.6
HSAs derived from the Huff model in Florida (β=1.43).

HSA yields the bed-to-population ratio, which can be used as a basic measure to depict the disparity in hospital resource allocation. Figure 5.7 indicates that lower bed-to-population ratios are found in larger HSAs, whereas higher bed-to-population ratios are around central city areas, such as Miami, Orlando, Jacksonville, and Pensacola.

Note that there are only 166 HSAs generated by the Huff model, which are 47 fewer than the 213 hospitals[6] in the study area. In other words, as estimated by the Huff model, those 47 hospitals are not visited by any ZIP code areas with the highest probability and thus do not have their own HSAs. For example, as shown in the inset of Figure 5.6, Jackson Memorial Hospital in Miami (with `Hosp _ ZoneID`=739) has 1,677 beds and outdraws other

---

[6] To be precise, there are 213 ZIP code areas with at least one hospital. See the data preparation in Section 1.3 in Chapter 1 for detail.

TABLE 5.1

HSAs Derived by the Huff Model in Florida

Distance Friction Coefficient	No. of HSAs	No. of HSAs without Hospitals	Population				Hospital Beds (for HSAs with Non-zero Beds)			
			Mean	Min	Max	Standard Deviation	Mean	Min	Max	Standard Deviation
$\beta=1$	118	6	159,349	78	3,058,700	370,327	507	25	6,303	743
$\beta=1.43$	166	11	113,272	3,662	2,076,116	217,021	366	15	3,732	443
$\beta=2$	185	9	101,639	1,475	1,526,759	145,428	322	15	3,128	356
$\beta=3$	196	9	95,935	6,297	955,720	99,639	303	8	3,078	337

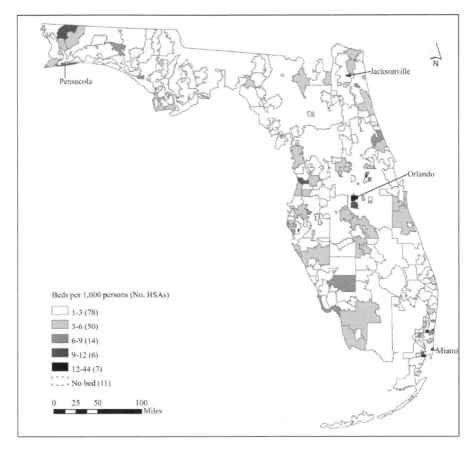

FIGURE 5.7
Bed sizes per 1,000 persons in HSAs derived by the Huff model (β=1.43).

surrounding hospitals in patient cares, even though some of those have large bed sizes such as 357 and 285 beds.

To further illustrate the important role of distance decay behavior in the Huff model, it is helpful to conduct a sensitivity analysis. Here we stay with the power function, but change the distance friction coefficient. When β=1, 2, and 3, the Huff model generates 118, 185, and 196 HSAs as shown in Figure 5.8a–c, respectively. Table 5.1 summarizes the population and hospital beds across HSAs by various distance friction coefficients. A larger distance friction coefficient leads to a higher number of HSAs. As β increases, the distance friction effect becomes stronger and patients value a closer hospital more; as a result, the derived HSAs become more fragmented and smaller. Reversely, when the β value decreases over time due to the improvements in transportation technologies or road network, travel distance matters to a less degree, giving even a stronger edge to larger and more comprehensive hospitals. This helps partially explain the consolidation of health market in the USA over time.

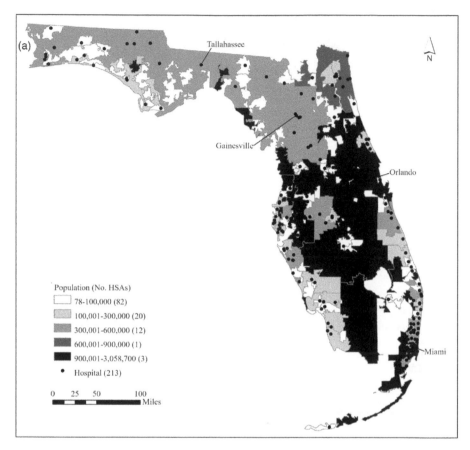

FIGURE 5.8
HSAs derived by the Huff model in Florida: (a) β=1, (b) β=2, and (c) β=3.   (*Continued*)

There remain two unresolved issues in the HSAs derived from the Huff model. Foremost, many HSAs are fragmented. In other words, an HSA may be composed of multiple areas that are not spatially contiguous. For example, as shown in Figure 5.9a, the HSA highlighted in shade is made of a large area on the north and four small areas in the southeast, and several smaller HSAs form enclaves within that large area. In addition, as it is the case in the afore-mentioned sensitivity analysis (Table 5.1), the Huff model sometimes yields HSAs without any hospitals inside. For example, as shown in Figure 5.9b, HSA 123 is composed of three ZIP code areas having the highest projected flows linking to one hospital, which is barely outside of its boundary, leading to no hospitals in the HSA. In comparison, either HSA 57 or HSA 64 has an anchor-ing hospital inside that draws the highest projected flows from surrounding ZIP code areas. Both issues have been accounted for in the refined Dartmouth method illustrated in Chapter 4. The following Section 5.4 will discuss the GIS automation of the Huff model and its post-treatment in addressing the issues.

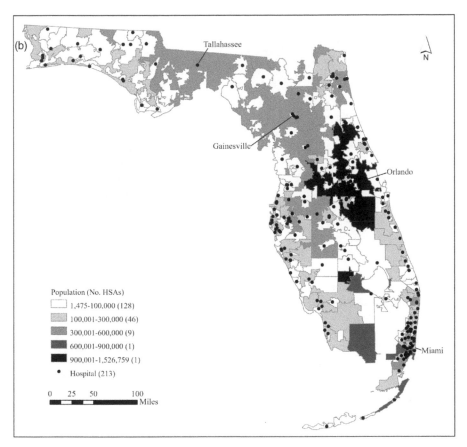

FIGURE 5.8 (Continued)
HSAs derived by the Huff model in Florida: (a) $\beta=1$, (b) $\beta=2$, and (c) $\beta=3$. (*Continued*)

5.4 Automated Delineation of HSAs by Integrating the Huff Model and Dartmouth Method

An improved toolkit of Huff Model Pro.tbx is developed in ArcGIS Pro to automate the implementation of the Huff model.[7] It includes two tools:

1. Huff model (based on Euclidean distances or geodesic distances between customers and facilities), and
2. Huff model with an external distance table.

---

[7] The subfolder Scripts contains the Python script for the toolkit. Be sure to copy the subfolder along with the file Huff Model Pro.tbx for the program to be executable.

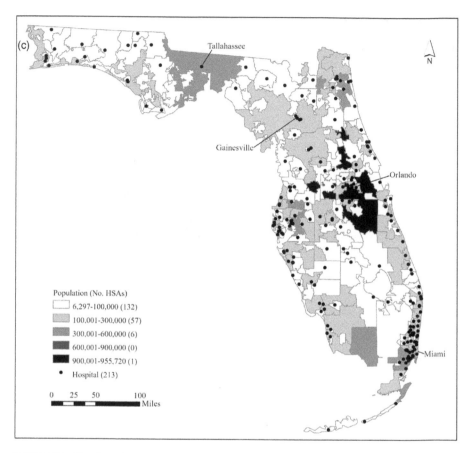

FIGURE 5.8 (Continued)
HSAs derived by the Huff model in Florida: (a) $\beta=1$, (b) $\beta=2$, and (c) $\beta=3$.

One may access the tools in ArcGIS Pro as follows: Under Catalog view, right-click Toolboxes, click Add Toolbox to select and add the toolkit Huff Model Pro.tbx, and expand the toolkit to display the two tools. See Figure 5.10a–b for the interfaces of the first tool "Huff Model", which calculates either Euclidean or geodesic distances between the supply and demand locations. If it is desirable to apply other measures of spatial impedance, one needs to prepare an external distance (or travel time) table beforehand and use the second tool "Huff Model w External Distance Table". See Figure 5.11 for its interface, which contains four items for defining the external distance table: table name, customer ID, facility ID, and travel impedance between them. The ID fields for customer and facility locations must be consistent with the corresponding layers and ID fields defined in the same interface. The second tool automates the step-by-step implementation of the Huff model in the case study illustrated in Section 5.3.

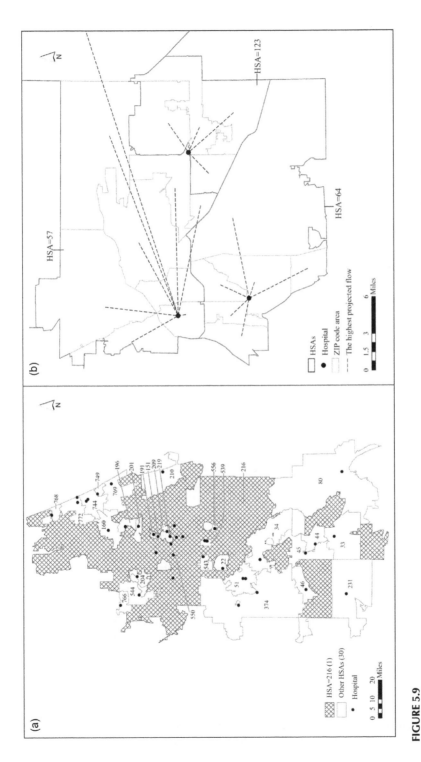

FIGURE 5.9
Problematic HSAs derived from the Huff model: (a) spatially non-contiguous HSA; (b) HSA without any hospitals inside.

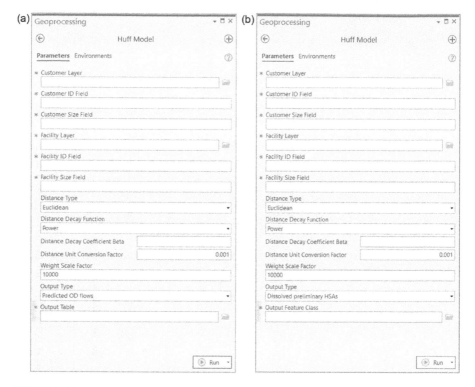

FIGURE 5.10
Interface for implementing the Huff model for (a) Predicted OD flows and (b) Dissolved preliminary HSAs.

Below is a quick overview of items to be defined in the two tools. Unless specified, the discussion applies to both tools:

- three items associated with the customer feature: layer name,[8] its unique ID field, and customer size (e.g., population),
- three items associated with the facility feature: layer name, its unique ID field, and facility size, which defines the variable *S* in Equation 5.6,
- for the first tool (Figure 5.10a and b), distance type which has two options "Euclidean" and "Geodesic" to choose from[9]; for the second tool (Figure 5.11), four items that are associated with the pre-defined distance (travel time) table: table name, customer ID, facility ID, and impedance values between them,

---

[8] If the desirable output is "Dissolved preliminary HSAs", the customer layer needs to be a polygon feature.

[9] If the customer feature class is defined in a geographic coordinate system, the tool automatically invokes the option of geodesic distance. If Euclidean distance is preferred, define a projected coordinate system for the customer feature.

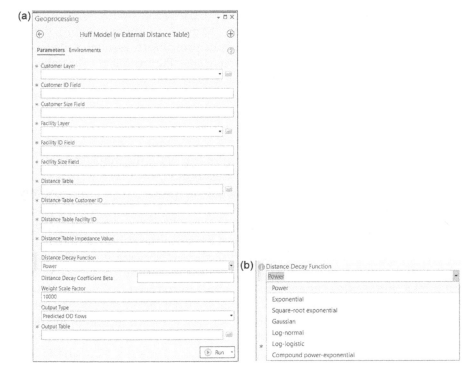

FIGURE 5.11
Interface for implementing the Huff model with an external distance table: (a) main window;
(b) sub-window for available choices of distance decay function.

- distance decay function $f(x)$, including one-parameter continuous functions (power, exponential, square-root exponential, Gaussian, and log-normal) or two-parameter continuous functions (log-logistic and compound power-exponential), and its associated coefficients[10] as discussed in Section 3.1,

- for the first tool (Figure 5.10a and b), distance unit conversion factor, with a default value of 0.001 (e.g., converting meters to kilometers),[11]

- weight scale factor for inflating the values for potentials, with a default value of 10,000 to avoid too small values, and finally

---

[10] The default values for the power, exponential, square-root exponential, and log-normal functions are set at 3, 0.03, 0.3, and 0.3, respectively. For the Gaussian function, the coefficient is the value for σ (with a default value = 80) since $\mu = 0$ for a monotonic distance decay pattern when assuming no crater around $x = 0$. The distance decay coefficient alpha appears only when a two-parameter function is chosen (Figure 5.10b). The default values for both parameters (alpha and beta) in the log-logistic and compound power-exponential functions are set at 1.

[11] Use of distance values in meters without conversion could be problematic especially for the exponential or Gaussian distance decay function, which is not scale independent. This option is not provided in the second tool.

- output type (associated table or feature class) for saving the results. When the option "Predicted OD flows" is chosen (default), the output is a table that includes fields of probability, estimated flows, and other fields related to the potentials (Figure 5.10a). The table could be used as an input for the Dartmouth method. When the option "Dissolved preliminary HSAs" is chosen, it generates a feature class that contains the dissolved HSAs with customer sizes from the customer feature (Figure 5.10b).

Before entering a value for each item, users can place the mouse on the red star next to the item to view its detailed description.

As stated previously, the Huff model is prone to derive spatially non-contiguous HSAs and some HSAs do not even contain any hospitals. The refined Dartmouth method illustrated in the Chapter 4 may help resolve these issues based on the estimated flows between the supply and demand locations from the Huff model. Figure 5.12 shows the parameter settings for the items when using the tool "Dartmouth Method (HSAs or HRRs)" under the toolkit of HSA Delineation Pro.tbx[12] introduced in Chapter 4. Item EstFlow is generated in step 3 in Section 5.3 or from the output table by using the aforementioned automated Huff model tool. For the delineation method, choose "Huff–Dartmouth Method" to delineate HSAs by the estimated flows from the Huff model. The spatial adjacency matrix, FLplgnAdjUp. npz, is generated by the tool of "Build A Spatial Adjacency Matrix" from step 1 in Sub-section 4.4.1. Leave Minimal Localization Index blank and default values for others. Name the Output Polygon Layer as HDHSAs under the FL _ HSA.gdb. Click Run, and the result will be loaded in the Map view.

Here the delineation method, "Huff–Dartmouth Method", extracts the maximum estimated flows from each of the ZIP code areas to start the process, whereas the other option "Dartmouth Method" discussed in Chapter 4 uses all actual flows. This strategy is adopted for improving the computational efficiency.[13] For a given number of demand sites (m) and a number of supply sites (n), the matrix of simulated flows between them is a complete $m \times n$ and sizable matrix, whereas the actual flow matrix is often a small fraction of that size. However, all estimated flows participate in the calculation of indices such as localization index (LI) and average travel time.

The Huff–Dartmouth method generates 113 continuous HSAs. Recall that the preliminary 166 HSAs derived from the Huff model in Section 5.3 have several problems such as non-contiguous HSAs and HSAs without containing any anchoring hospitals inside. Those preliminary HSAs are adjusted

---

[12] As mentioned in Chapter 4, this toolkit relies on some Python packages. For the first-time users, we refer them to follow the instructions in Section 4.3 to clone the Python environment in ArcGIS Pro and install the required Python packages.

[13] On a desktop PC of Intel(R) Xeon(R) Gold 6140 CPU @ 2.30GHz with 128GB RAM, it takes 23 seconds for preserving only the maximum flows, while it needs 3.8 minutes if all estimated flows are used.

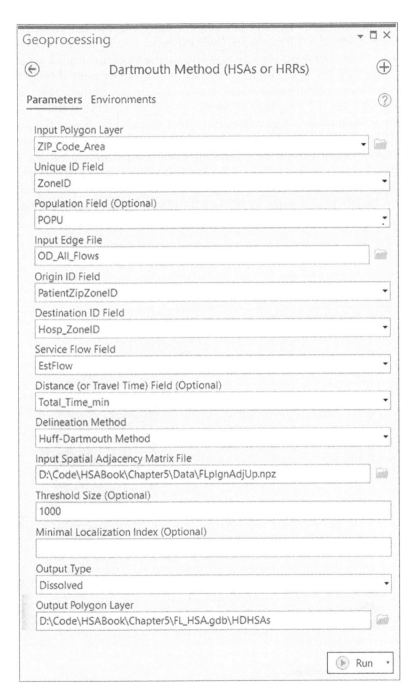

FIGURE 5.12
Interface of parameter settings for Huff–Dartmouth-derived HSAs in Florida.

and consolidated into the 113 HSAs by employing the automated Huff–
Dartmouth method, which essentially is the refined Dartmouth method and
addresses these problems. Figure 5.13 shows the variations of LI across 113
HSAs. Note that the so-called LIs are calculated from estimated hospitalization flows from the Huff model and have relatively low values. The majority
of HSAs have LI<0.3. The Huff model is a simple model that relies only on
the simple assumption of gravitational effect dictated by hospital sizes and
travel times between hospitals and residents, and understandably its estimated flow pattern cannot be taken as a perfect replacement for the actual
flow data. In the absence of hospitalization flow data, the Huff model offers
us an opportunity to develop a preliminary configuration of hospital care
markets. Reliable delineation of HSAs still relies on actual patient visit data.

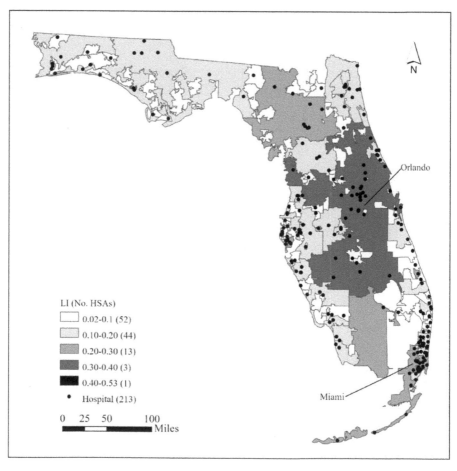

FIGURE 5.13
Localization index values and hospitals in 113 Huff–Dartmouth derived HSAs.

Lack of data for specialized care capacities in hospitals[14] prevents us from exploring the delineation of HRRs based on the Huff model. The result from the Huff model is also derived under very different data requirements from what is needed for implementing the refined Dartmouth method in Chapter 4 and the network community detection methods in Chapter 6. Therefore, no comparisons or discussion on their results are made.

5.5 Summary

This chapter introduced the proximal area method and the Huff model for delineating HSAs. The proximal area method simply assumes that patients use their nearest hospitals and thus defines an HSA made of areas sharing the same nearest hospital. The Huff model estimates the probabilities of patients choosing hospitals based on a gravity model, which accounts for the joint effects of hospital sizes and distances between the patients' residences and hospitals. In other words, the Huff model estimates the hospitalization service flow pattern and uses the plurality rule like the Dartmouth method in Chapter 4 to define HSAs.

The proximal area method is implemented by utilizing several tools in ArcGIS corresponding to the distance or travel time measures. The Huff model is first illustrated by a step-by-step implementation in ArcGIS Pro to help readers develop an in-depth understanding of the model's formulation. The process is then automated in a toolkit of two options: (1) computing the Euclidean or geodesic distance internally and completing the model calibration in one tool, or (2) reading a pre-defined distance matrix to implement the model in another tool. Both offer the choice of obtaining a table of estimated patient OD flows or deriving the dissolved HSAs. The derived HSAs may be spatially non-contiguous or miss anchoring hospitals inside HSAs and require post-treatment that is accomplished by using an automated tool similar to the refined Dartmouth method introduced in Chapter 4.

While the concepts of proximal area method and the Huff model are straightforward, their successful implementation relies on adequate measurements of variables including travel impedance. As discussed in Chapter 2, travel impedance measures go beyond distance or travel time and vary by transportation modes. Travel cost, convenience, comfort, or safety may also be important. People from various socioeconomic or demographic groups and in different geographic areas may experience spatial impedance differently. Accounting for interactions by telecommunication, Internet, and other

---

[14] The data discussed in Section 1.3 include total bed sizes for specialized hospitals, but do not specify how much portion is dedicated to specialized cares such as cardiovascular surgery and neurosurgery.

modern technologies adds further complexity to the issue. This chapter is limited to the technical implementation of related GIS methods.

Why do we need to estimate the flows by the Huff model while we already have the data of actual flows? The answer is no. However, such information, like other medical data, is often unavailable, and the use of the Huff model becomes necessary. More importantly, the model helps us predict the impact of changes in a health care market such as opening of new hospitals, and closing, expansion, downscaling, or relocation of the existing ones.

6

Delineating Hospital Service Areas by Network Community Detection Methods

The two preceding chapters discuss two methods for delineating hospital service areas (HSAs). Chapter 4 introduces the refined Dartmouth method that utilizes an existing patient service flow dataset between residences of patients and hospitals. In the absence of such an actual hospital utilization dataset, Chapter 5 relies on the Huff model to interpolate the hospitalization pattern. Both employ a plurality rule to assign areas (e.g., ZIP code areas) to hospitals being visited most often, and then areas assigned to the same hospital form its HSA. However, the plurality rule cannot guarantee that residents use most services within the defined HSA as each assignment only considers the greatest proportion of patients to one hospital at a time. In other words, it lacks a systematic perspective of ensuring the maximal total service volume within derived HSAs.

This chapter introduces the network community detection approach, considered the most promising technique for HSA delineation that has been available only recently. It follows a simple principle of grouping what is linked while keeping apart what is not (Reichardt and Bornholdt, 2006). As a result, HSAs are formed by grouping most densely interconnected areas in terms of service volumes. The maximal service volumes within the HSAs, while minimal between them, are achieved by innovative network community detection methods.

Section 6.1 discusses two network community detection methods, namely the Louvain and Leiden algorithms. The Louvain algorithm, one of the most popular and high-performing algorithms, is chosen as a baseline, and the very recent Leiden algorithm has shown some advantages in our pilot study. Section 6.2 illustrates how the two algorithms are refined to account for some spatial properties required or desirable for HSA delineation, termed spatially constrained Louvain and Leiden methods (or simply "ScLouvain" and "ScLeiden"). Section 6.3 uses the automated tools for ScLouvain and ScLeiden to delineate HSAs and HRRs in Florida. Section 6.4 evaluates the performances by comparing the two network community detection methods as well as against the refined Dartmouth method. Section 6.5 concludes the chapter with a summary.

DOI: 10.1201/9780429260285-6

6.1 Community Detection Methods: From Louvain to Leiden

While the Dartmouth method and Huff model group small areas to form HSAs by emphasizing the greatest proportion of patient visits (i.e., the plurality rule), community detection in network analysis considers almost all patient visits to hospitals. Based on a network of hospitalization patterns between nodes (e.g., ZIP code areas), *community detection* groups nodes with dense connections into initial communities and continues to group dense connections between initial communities into higher-level communities until a single community for a whole study area is attained. The process is guided by maximizing a quality measure, "modularity", for detected communities and generates a series of HSAs where lower-level (smaller) HSAs are nested within higher-level (larger) HSAs.

The work by Hu et al. (2018) is among the first in applying the approach to delineate HSAs by adopting the popular *"Louvain algorithm"* (Blondel et al., 2008, named after the University of Louvain, with which the authors are affiliated)[1]. Wang et al. (2020) also used the Louvain algorithm in delineating cancer service areas (CSAs) in the Northeast Region of the USA. One deficiency of the Louvain algorithm is its tendency to generate arbitrarily poorly connected or even internally disconnected communities when iteratively running it. Motivated by providing a remedy to this deficiency, Traag et al. (2019) proposed the *"Leiden algorithm"* (named after Leiden University, with which the research team is affiliated)[2], which guarantees connected communities and is computationally more efficient. This section discusses both the algorithms.

Modularity is one of the best-known quality measures in community detection studies (Newman, 2004; Newman and Girvan, 2004). It compares the total number of edges (or total weights of edges for a weighted network) that fall within all communities in a network to that in a null model (i.e., random network). Community detection maximizes the difference between the actual number of flows within each community and the expected number of such flows by chance (random). The resulting flows within each community are then more tightly connected with each other, while the inter-community flows are sparsely connected. For an undirected and weighted network, modularity is given by incorporating a tunable resolution parameter:

$$Q = \sum_{c \in C} \left(\frac{l_{in}^c}{m} - \gamma \left(\frac{k_{tot}^c}{2m} \right)^2 \right) \tag{6.1}$$

---

[1] According to the Google Scholar dated July 26, 2021, the paper by Blondel et al. (2008) has been cited 14,773 times.

[2] According to the Google Scholar dated July 26, 2021, the paper by Traag et al. (2019) has already been cited 628 times.

where Q represents the modularity value that sums over each community $c \in C$, l_{in}^c is the total number of edge weights between all nodes within community c, k_{tot}^c is the sum of the edge weights between nodes in community c and nodes in other communities, and m is the total number of edge weights in the network. In Equation 6.1, the first term $\dfrac{l_{in}^c}{m}$ represents the fraction of the sum of the edge weights in community c and the second term $\dfrac{k_{tot}^c}{2m}$ represents the expected fraction of edge weights between different communities. Therefore, maximizing the modularity is to maximize the difference between the two terms and thus simultaneously maximize the intra-community edge weights while minimizing the inter-community edge weights. The constant $\gamma > 0$ is the resolution parameter, and a higher resolution γ leads to a larger number of communities. Generally, a higher modularity value represents higher-quality communities and thus a more stable and robust network structure.

Based on Equation 6.1, the local gain of modularity of moving (grouping) a node i to a community c, denoted by $\Delta Q_{i \to c}$, is simplified as:

$$\Delta Q_{i \to c} = \frac{1}{m} \left(k_{i,in} - \gamma \frac{k_i * \Sigma_{total}}{2m} \right) \tag{6.2}$$

where $\gamma > 0$ remains the resolution parameter, m is the total number of edge weights in the network, $k_{i, in}$ is the sum of edge weights from node i to nodes in community c, k_i is the sum of edge weights linked to node i, and Σ_{total} is the sum of edge weights linked to nodes in community c.

The Louvain algorithm is a popular, elegant, and high-performing technique for modularity optimization (Blondel et al., 2008). It has two phases: (1) local nodes moving and (2) network aggregation. The local nodes moving phase begins with treating each node of the network as a unique community, and then removes each node from its original community to different communities temporarily and finds the community for which the local gain of modularity in Equation 6.2 is maximal. If the community is detected, the move becomes permanent; otherwise, the node returns to its original community. The process iterates across all nodes until no further improvement of modularity is possible. The network aggregation phase starts from constructing a new network by aggregating communities in the local nodes moving phase to become new nodes and updating the edge weights. It then repeats the first phase until obtaining a single community or no further improvement of modularity. This bottom-up process builds communities of communities iteratively and yields a hierarchy. Each level has a local optimum of modularity, and its level corresponds to the iteration of the first phase.

As Traag et al. (2019) discovered, the Louvain algorithm heavily relies on a single indicator, modularity, to measure the quality of network partition and tends to yield poorly connected or even disconnected communities. In the first phase, all nodes are eventually moved to an expected community. If a node happens to be a network hub and moving it to a new community achieves the maximal gain of modularity, the node may still act as a virtual bridge between other nodes in the old community. If other nodes are strongly connected to the old community like sub-communities, removing such a node will disconnect the old community. In other words, the local nodes move may cause globally disconnected communities.

Traag et al. (2019) proposed the Leiden algorithm to remedy the drawback of the Louvain algorithm and to guarantee communities well connected with a higher computational efficiency. The Leiden algorithm consists of three phases: (1) local nodes moving, (2) refinement of the partition, and (3) network aggregation based on the refinement, but using the non-refined partition to initialize the aggregated network. For the first phase, unlike the Louvain algorithm that keeps moving all nodes, the Leiden algorithm employs the *fast local move* procedure (Bae et al., 2017; Ozaki et al., 2016) to only visit those whose neighboring communities have changed. In short, the fast local move procedure randomly loads all nodes of the network into a queue, and then moves the first node from the front of the queue to different communities and detects the one for which the local positive gain of modularity is maximal. The node's neighbors that are neither in the new community nor in the queue are added to the rear of the queue. Such steps continue until the queue is empty. In this way, the Leiden algorithm is more efficient than the Louvain algorithm. In the second phase of refinement, the Leiden algorithm uses the *smart local move* (Waltman and Van Eck, 2013) to detect well-connected subnetworks in each community and aims to provide more room to split them for high-quality partition. Specifically, it treats each community from the first phase as a subnetwork. In each subnetwork, it assigns each node to a community and only considers those well connected within the subnetwork. It then uses the *random neighbor move* to identify any community that increases the modularity rather than maxima, which allows a broader exploration in the partition space. This process iterates until all communities from the first phase are visited. As a result, some communities may be split into sub-communities while others remain intact. Therefore, the Leiden algorithm resolves any poorly connected or disconnected communities.

The proposition of the Leiden algorithm was motivated by mitigating some of the problems associated with the Louvain algorithm. However, there is no guarantee that the Leiden algorithm outperforms the Louvain algorithm in all applications (Traag et al. 2019, p. 8). The Leiden algorithm is just new, and a full validation of its advantages awaits as more applications are implemented in various fields.

6.2 Spatially Constrained Louvain and Leiden Methods

Adopting the community detection methods such as the Louvain and Leiden algorithms for delineating HSAs needs to account for spatial constraints, foremost to ensure that the derived service areas are spatially contiguous. There are other constraints, for example, a threshold population size (e.g., 120,000 for HRRs by the Dartmouth method). More recently, C Wang et al. (2021a) have built upon these two community detection algorithms and developed their spatially constrained versions, termed *"spatially constrained Louvain (ScLouvain)"* and *"spatially constrained Leiden (ScLeiden)"* methods, for delineating the CSAs in the Northeast Region of the USA. This section illustrates the specific steps to implement the ScLouvain and ScLeiden methods.

The ScLouvain method has three steps: (1) local nodes moving, (2) network aggregation, and (3) spatial contiguity and minimal region size guarantees. The ScLeiden method contains four phases: (1) local nodes moving, (2) refinement, (3) network aggregation based on the refined partition, and (4) spatial contiguity and minimal region size guarantees. The last step in both the methods is added to the original algorithms to make them spatially constrained.

Figures 6.1 and 6.2 illustrate the implementation of the ScLouvain and ScLeiden methods, respectively, to aggregate 19 nodes in a simple network to three communities. In our case study that follows in Section 6.3, both patients and hospitals are consolidated into ZIP code areas. The nodes represent the ZIP code areas of patients or the ZIP code areas of facilities or both. The edge weights are service flow volumes between the nodes in both directions. As shown in Figures 6.1a and 6.2a, the 19 nodes indexed as 1–19 in circles represent the locations of patients or hospitals in 19 ZIP code areas (polygons with boundaries in light gray). The dark lines labeled with numbers represent the service flow volumes of edges between nodes. The network has all nodes connected, but node 19 at the lower-left corner unconnected.

In the nodes moving phase, both the ScLouvain and ScLeiden methods begin with assigning 19 nodes to 19 individual communities (Figures 6.1a and 6.2a). Then the ScLouvain method repeatedly moves each individual node to different communities and identifies the community for which the positive gain of local modularity is greatest. This process continues until there is no further improvement of modularity at the current level. Eventually, it detects five communities in terms of the entire network and each community contains the same color polygons in Figure 6.1b. In contrast, the ScLeiden method uses the fast local move procedure to speed up the process as there may exist unnecessary movements of nodes. Some nodes may still stay in their original community after a series of move-in and move-out operations. As shown in Figure 6.2b, the ScLeiden method

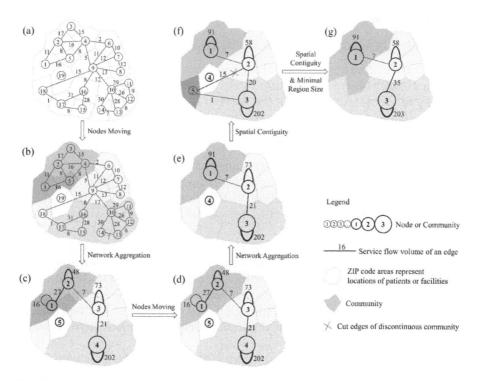

FIGURE 6.1
Schematic illustration of ScLouvain method.

also derives five communities represented by five different gray levels when the partition is stable. Note that two separate sets of nodes: (15, 16, and 17) at the bottom middle and (10, 11, 12, 13, and 14) at the bottom right, belong to the highlighted community in terms of the entire network, but they are two sub-communities in terms of the local subnetworks. This is attributable to the role of node 9 acting as a bridge to connect two sub-communities. It is later moved to the community composed of nodes (6, 7, and 8) for gaining modularity, leaving two sub-communities internally disconnected. Node 9 also has a strong connection with a non-adjacent node 18 at the lower left, which is assigned to the same community for the greatest modularity gain.

Next, the ScLouvain method creates a new network, where five communities become five new nodes (to be renumbered) and the service volumes between any new nodes are updated (see Figure 6.1c). However, the ScLeiden method adopts the smart local move and the random neighbor move to refine the five communities by splitting the highlighted community into two sub-communities, in which a set of nodes (15, 16, and 17) and another set of nodes (10, 11, 12, 13, and 14) are well connected, respectively (see Figure 6.2c). This is a significant difference between the two methods. The ScLeiden

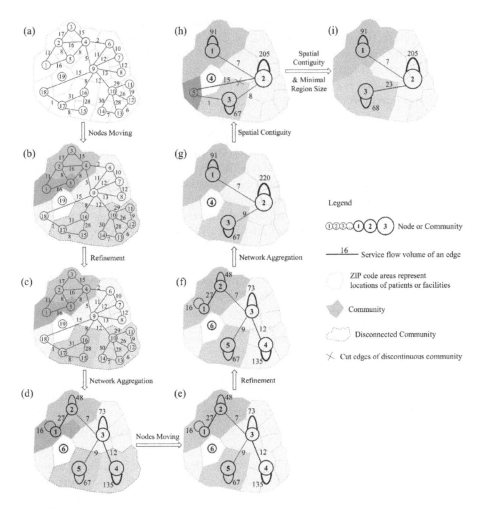

FIGURE 6.2
Schematic illustration of ScLeiden method.

method uses the non-refined partition to initialize the aggregated network in order to guarantee the monotonically increasing modularity[3] and still yields five communities but with the highlighted community locally separated into two sub-communities (two polygons in different gray levels at the bottom in Figure 6.2d).

Then both methods start the second iteration. Since nodes 1 and 2 at the top-left corner have strong connections with each other, both methods move

---

[3] Although the poorly connected communities detected in this phase have small edge weights between nodes in each community, having one big community in the aggregated network will have modularity higher than that derived from multiple sub-communities detected in the refinement phase.

them into one community for the greatest modularity gain in the local nodes moving phase (Figures 6.1d and 6.2e). The ScLeiden method even moves node 4 at the lower right corner to the node 3 community to maximize the modularity gain (Figure 6.2e). The ScLouvain method continues to aggregate the network to one with four new nodes (Figure 6.1e). The ScLeiden method refines the partition (Figure 6.2f) and aggregates the network to a different one with four new nodes (Figure 6.2g). Both methods obtain the best aspatial community structure with no further improvement of modularity.

The final phase is to enforce the spatial contiguity and minimal region size rules. Based on a pre-defined spatial adjacency matrix, we split the communities of the aspatial network that are not spatially contiguous (e.g., orphan, enclaved, or enclosed nodes). For example, the community represented by node 2 in Figure 6.1e or 6.2g is separated into two communities represented by node 5 and node 2 that are not adjacent in Figure 6.1f or 6.2h. Both methods yield five communities (nodes) at the cost of decreasing modularity as we split four into five communities.

To be consistent with the original definition of HSAs, each node (or HSA) should have a population size above the threshold and contain at least one hospital (or one destination node here). Otherwise, further aggregation is needed to account for the following scenarios:

1. For an *orphan node* with no edges (zero service volume) to any nodes in the network (neither an internal edge to itself nor outgoing edges to others), merge the node to its neighboring node (or HSA) with at least one hospital and the smallest population size (e.g., node 4 in Figures 6.1f and 6.2h is moved to node 1 and node 3 in Figures 6.1g and 6.2i, respectively).

2. For an *enclaved node* with or without edges connecting to its adjacent neighboring nodes but having edges connecting to multiple non-adjacent nodes, merge it to the adjacent neighboring node that achieves the maximal modularity gain, and if there is no positive gain in modularity, merge it to the adjacent neighboring node with hospitals and the smallest population size (e.g., the lower-left node 5 in Figures 6.1f and 6.2h is moved to node 3 in Figures 6.1g and 6.2i, respectively);

3. For an *enclosed node* with one neighboring node like a hole in a donut HSA, merge it directly to its neighbor.

This process continues until each community has a minimal regional size and at least one hospital when a global optimal modularity is achieved. Eventually, both methods aggregate the ZIP code areas to three contiguous service areas so that the total edge weights are maximal within the derived areas and minimal between them (Figures 6.1g and 6.2i). Note that the service areas represented by nodes 2 and 3 are different by the two methods as the ScLeiden method can identify poorly or disconnected communities and refine them.

Based on our experiences, the Leiden algorithm is likely to outperform the Louvain algorithm in most cases but not necessarily always. Enforcing the spatial constraints introduces further complexity to the process,[4] especially in the network aggregation phase. It is important to assess on a case-by-case basis whether the expected advantages in one algorithm over the other are materialized in their spatialized counterparts.

6.3 Automated Delineation of HSAs and HRRs and a Case Study in Florida

6.3.1 Automating the ScLouvain and ScLeiden Methods in ArcGIS Pro

The ScLouvain and ScLeiden methods are implemented in a tool "Network Community Detection Method (ScLeiden or ScLouvain)" under the toolkit of HSA Delineation Pro.tbx in ArcGIS Pro. After adding the toolkit to Toolboxes under the Project in Contents pane, right-click the tool of "Network Community Detection Method (ScLeiden or ScLouvain)" and select Properties to open the dialog window of Tool Properties. In General tab, verify the path of Script File pointing to the same Python script under the folder Scripts.

As shown in Figure 6.3, the tool has the following items to define:

- Three items associated with the input polygon feature: the polygon layer, its unique ID field, and the optional population field. The input polygon feature should have a projected coordinate system to ensure the index of geographic compactness is calibrated properly.

- Five items associated with the input flow network data: the input edge file, its origin ID field, destination ID field, service flow field and distance (or travel time) field between the two. Both the origin ID field and the destination ID field are unique and correspond to the unique ID field in the input polygon layer. The distance (or travel time) field is optional.

- Delineation method: choose the ScLouvain method or the ScLeiden method.

---

[4] The current versions of ScLouvain and ScLeiden do not yet account for a constraint of minimum localization index (LI).

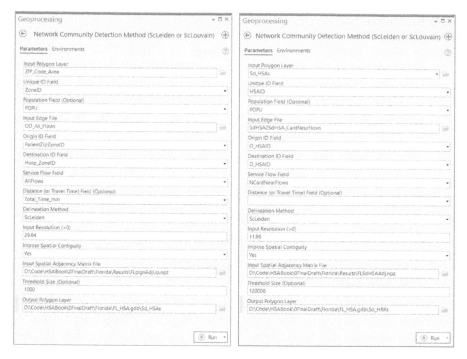

FIGURE 6.3
Interface for delineating (a) 136 HSAs and (b) 58 HRRs by the ScLeiden method.

- Input resolution (>0) that refers to the resolution parameter value of γ in Equation 6.1, with a default value of 1 that usually corresponds to the scenario with the global maximal modularity. As an important property of the network community detection method, users can change this value to delineate different numbers of communities.

- Three items associated with imposing spatial constraints: impose spatial contiguity (with options "Yes" and "No"), input spatial adjacency matrix file,[5] and threshold size (optional). When choosing "Yes" to impose spatial contiguity, users need to prepare a spatial adjacency matrix in advance. See Section 4.3 in Chapter 4 on how to use the tool "Build A Spatial Adjacency Matrix". When choosing "No", the task is to generate aspatial communities without imposing any spatial constraints, and the interface will not display the item "Input Spatial Adjacency Matrix" or "Threshold Size (Optional)". Threshold size refers to population size of each derived community, with a suggested default value of 1,000 for defining HSAs. Note that the usage of the threshold size requires a field containing the population data.

---

[5] The spatial adjacency matrix file must end with ".npz" format as discussed in Chapter 4. If the file browse on the right side of the item does not work for loading the ".npz" file, users need to copy the full path of the spatial adjacency matrix file to the corresponding item in the tool.

- Output polygon layer for saving the results. The output polygon layer is dissolved from the input polygon layer. Several indices introduced in Sub-section 4.4.2 of Chapter 4 are calculated, such as the localization index (LI), geographic compactness, and population size. Under the same path, there is a non-dissolved polygon layer with an extended name "NotDis" to record the relationship between the input polygon feature and the delineated communities.

After running this tool, two options, "View Details" and "Open History", are shown at the bottom of the dialog window. Users can click "View Details" and expand the Messages to review detailed information about the network and the modularity of the delineation result.

In summary, this tool can be applied in four scenarios by adjusting resolution values and threshold sizes to generate a series of communities (i.e., HSAs or HRRs) for various research purposes. That is,

1. generate aspatial communities without any spatial constraints in a non-dissolved layer,
2. generate aspatial communities without any spatial constraints in a dissolved layer with several indices,
3. generate spatial communities in a non-dissolved layer to record the relationship between the input feature and derived communities, and
4. generate spatial communities in a dissolved layer to evaluate the quality of the method by comparing different indices.

6.3.2 Delineating HSAs and HRRs in Florida by the ScLouvain and ScLeiden Methods

Similar to Chapter 4, this case study also uses the feature class ZIP _ Code _ Area, two tables OD _ All _ Flows and OD _ CardNeur _ Flows under FL _ HSA.gdb to delineate HSAs and HRRs in Florida by the ScLouvain and ScLeiden methods. A workflow is illustrated in Figure 6.4 to show the process of delineating two types of HSAs and two types of HRRs by the ScLeiden method. A similar workflow applies to the ScLouvain method. Using the feature layer ZIP _ Code _ Area and table OD _ All _ Flows, the ScLeiden method derives 18 HSAs with a global optimal modularity and 136 Dartmouth comparable HSAs discussed in Chapter 4. Using the 136 newly derived HSAs and the table OD _ CardNeur _ Flows, the ScLeiden method delineates 20 HRRs with a global optimal modularity and 58 Dartmouth comparable HRRs.

In ArcGIS Pro, under Catalog view, right-click Toolboxes and click Add Toolbox to open the dialog window, select and add the toolkit of "HSA Delineation Pro.tbx" from the data folder Florida. Expand

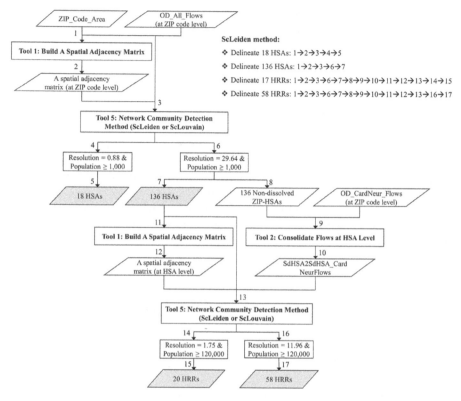

FIGURE 6.4
Workflow of using three tools to delineate HSAs and HRRs by the ScLeiden method.

the toolkit to display five tools. This case study uses three tools, "Build A Spatial Adjacency Matrix", "Consolidate Flows at HSA Level", and "Network Community Detection Method (ScLeiden or ScLouvain)".

As mentioned in Chapter 4, this toolkit relies on some Python packages. First-time users refer Section 4.3 in Chapter 4 and follow the instructions to clone a Python environment in ArcGIS Pro and install the required Python packages.

We firstly illustrate how to use the toolkit "HSA Delineation Pro.tbx" to delineate 136 HSAs by the ScLeiden method in Florida.

1. Use the tool "Build A Spatial Adjacency Matrix".

   This step is identical to the first step of delineating HSAs in Sub-section 4.4.1. Skip the step if users have already generated a spatial adjacency matrix file between the ZIP code areas. The parameter settings are shown in Figure 4.4a in Chapter 4. Select ZIP_Code_Area for Input Polygon Layer and ZoneID for Unique ID Field, choose "Yes" for Adjusted, and select the appended spatial adjacency matrix "FLplgnAdjAppend.csv" to account for ZIP code areas that are separated by natural barriers but are connected via a physical road network. Select the path and name the output file as "FLplgnAdjUp.npz". Click Run.

2. Use the tool "Network Community Detection Method (ScLeiden or ScLouvain)".

As shown in Figure 6.3a, select the feature class ZIP _ Code _ Area for Input Polygon Layer, ZoneID for Unique ID Field, and POPU for Population Field. Select the table OD _ All _ Flows under the same geodatabase for Input Edge File, PatientZipZoneID for Origin ID Field, Hosp _ ZoneID for Destination ID Field, AllFlows for Service Flow Field, and Total _ Time _ min for Distance (or Travel Time) Field. Choose ScLeiden for Delineation Method, and input 29.64[6] for Input Resolution. Choose "Yes" for Impose Spatial Contiguity. Select "FLplgnAdjUp.npz" for Input Spatial Adjacency Matrix File. Leave Threshold Size as default value of 1,000. Give the name "Sd _ HSAs" for Output Polygon Layer. Click Run.

The feature class Sd _ HSAs has 136 spatially contiguous HSAs. Open its attribute table. It has field HSAID to identify each HSA, field COUNT _ ZoneID to record the number of ZIP code areas, field Num _ DZoneID for the number of destination ZIP code areas (or hospitals) within each HSA, and four additional fields LI, POPU, Compactness, and EstTime to represent the localization index, population size, geographic compactness, and average travel time of each HSA. The definition of each index is given in Sub-section 4.4.2 of Chapter 4. The non-dissolved feature class Sd _ HSAsNotDis is also generated under the same path to record the relationship between ZIP code areas and HSAs.

If users want to generate HSAs with a global optimal modularity based on the ScLeiden method, input an appropriate value, such as 0.88, for Input Resolution, change the name of the output polygon layer, and leave others as the above settings. Click Run again to generate a new set of HSAs.

The automated delineation of HRRs is similar, but has one more step. Recall that the HRRs are made of whole HSAs, and the cardiovascular surgery and neurosurgery flow data are provided at the ZIP code level and need to be consolidated at the HSA level. This is different from the work reported in Hu et al. (2018), which used the cardiovascular surgery and neurosurgery flows at the ZIP code level to directly construct HRRs. The following steps illustrate how to define 59 HRRs based on the 136 HSAs by the ScLeiden method. The same toolkit is used.

1. Use the tool "Consolidate Flows at HSA Level"

As shown in Figure 6.5, select the table OD _ CardNeur _ Flows for Input Edge File, PatientZipZoneID for Origin ID Field,

---

[6] Because of the random order in node movement in the two network community detection methods, users may need to slightly adjust the resolution value or run multiple times to reach 136 HSAs.

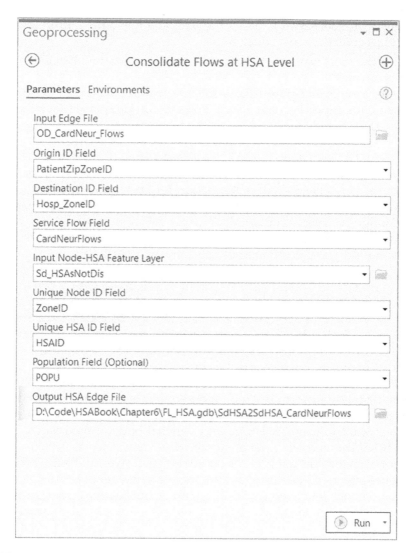

FIGURE 6.5
Interface for consolidating cardiovascular surgery and neurosurgery flows at the ZIP code level to the ScLeiden-derived HSA level.

Hosp _ ZoneID for Destination ID Field, and CardNeurFlows for Service Flow Field. Select the pre-defined feature class Sd _ HSAsNotDis for Input Node-HSA Feature Layer, and select ZoneID for Unique Node ID Field, HSAID for Unique HSA ID Field, and POPU for Population Field. Name the Output HSA Edge File as a table SdHSA2SdHSA _ CardNeurFlows. Click Run to consolidate the cardiovascular surgery and neurosurgery flows between ZIP codes areas to flows between HSAs.

The new table has 4,576 records with a total volume of 293,050, identical to the total service volumes from the table OD _ CardNeur _ Flows. Open the attribute table. It has four fields O _ HSAID, D _ HSAID, NCardNeurFlows, and Num _ DZoneID to represent the origin HSAID, destination HSAID, total service volumes between the two, and the number of destination ZIP code areas (or hospitals) within the destination HSA. Ensure that the name of the field Num _ DZoneID remains unchanged, and it will be used to calculate the total number of destination ZIP codes within each HRR.

2. Use the tool "Build A Spatial Adjacency Matrix"

As shown in Figure 6.6, select the previously dissolved HSAs feature class Sd _ HSAs for Input Polygon Layer, choose HSAID for Unique ID Field, leave Adjusted as default value "No", and name the Output File as FLSdHSAAdj.npz under a folder rather than in a geodatabase. Click Run to generate a spatial adjacency matrix between HSAs, saved as a csv file under the same path. Note that the csv file only contains the ZIP code pairs that are adjacent. Users can use it

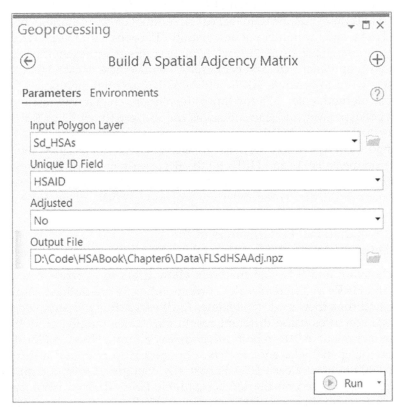

FIGURE 6.6
Building a spatial adjacency matrix from 136 HSAs derived from the ScLeiden method.

to generate a flow map to verify that all HSAs are spatially adjacent based on the queen contiguity rule.

3. Use the tool "Network Community Detection Method (ScLeiden or ScLouvain)"

As shown in Figure 6.3b, select Sd _ HSAs for Input Polygon Layer, HSAID for Unique ID field, and POPU for Population Field. Select the table SdHSA2SdHSA _ CardNeurFlows derived from step 1 for Input Edge File, O _ HSAID for Origin ID Field, D _ HSAID for Destination ID Field, and NCardNeurFlows for Service Flow Field. Leave the Distance (or Travel Time) Field blank. Select ScLeiden for Delineation Method, and input 11.96 for Resolution. Select "Yes" for Impose Spatial Contiguity and FLSdHSAAdj.npz from step 2 for Input Spatial Adjacency Matrix File. Input 120,000 for Threshold Size. Name Output Polygon Layer as Sd _ HRRs. Click Run.

The feature class Sd _ HRRs has 58 spatially contiguous HRRs, and each HRR has a population size greater than 120,000. Open the attribute table. It has a field HRRID to identify each HRR, three fields COUNT _ HSAID, Num _ DHSAID, and Num _ DZoneID to record the number of HSAs, number of destination HSAs, and the number of destination ZIP codes within each HRR, and three additional fields LI, POPU, and Compactness to represent the localization index, population size, and geographic compactness of each HRR.

If users want to generate HRRs with a global optimal modularity by the ScLeiden method, enter 1.75 for Input Resolution, change the name of the output polygon layer, and leave others as the above settings. Click Run again to generate a new set of HRRs.

Change the Delineation Method to "ScLouvain", and repeat the same steps to delineate HSAs and HRRs by the ScLouvain method. The suggested resolution values are 1.38 and 30.23 for deriving 22 and 136 HSAs, respectively, and are 1.75 and 11.96 for deriving 22 and 59 HRRs, respectively.

6.3.3 Computational Performances of the ScLouvain and ScLeiden Methods

The ScLouvain and ScLeiden methods allow users to generate a series of HSAs and HRRs at different scales corresponding to pre-defined resolution values, and thus they are scale-flexible. To illustrate this property, we simulate 1,000 scenarios using different resolution values ranging from 0 to 10 with an increment of 0.01 in both methods to delineate HSAs in Florida. We also use the spatial adjacency matrix, FLplgnAdjUp.npz, and a threshold size of 1,000 to ensure each HSA is spatially contiguous with a population size over 1,000. Based on the 136 comparable HSAs derived from the two methods, we also simulate 1,500 scenarios of HRRs based on the cardiovascular surgery and neurosurgery flows with resolution values ranging from 0 to 15 with an increment of 0.01 for both methods. The spatial adjacency matrix derived for the 136 HSAs and a threshold size of 120,000 are also used for defining the HRRs. Both the algorithms are very efficient and complete each round of simulation in a fraction of minute[7].

Figure 6.7a shows that the trend lines of modularity versus the number of HSAs from the ScLouvain and ScLeiden methods are largely consistent. Figure 6.7b shows that the trend lines for the aspatial Louvain and Leiden methods (i.e., without imposing the spatial constraints) are much more consistent across scales. For the same number of HSAs, there are multiple modularity values corresponding to different resolution values with small increments. Overall, all exhibit a right-tail normal distribution. Similar numbers of HSAs derived from the ScLouvain and ScLeiden methods have lower modularity values than their predecessors, respectively. For example, the ScLouvain method delineates 22 HSAs with a modularity value of 0.8456 in Figure 6.7a, lower than 0.8458 of the 21 HSAs derived from the Louvain method in Figure 6.7b. The same applies to the ScLeiden and Leiden methods (0.8443 for 18 ScLeiden HSAs vs. 0.8463 for 19 Leiden HSAs). A few scenarios in the middle of Figure 6.7a have significantly different modularity values by the two methods. This is mainly attributable to different impacts of two constraints added to the ScLouvain and ScLeiden methods. The enforcement of spatial contiguity splits non-contiguous HSAs at the cost of decreasing modularity, while ensuring the minimal region size enables the merger of smaller HSAs to larger ones and results in an increase in modularity. The two methods also yield different numbers of global optimal HSAs. As shown in Figure 6.7a, the ScLouvain method yields the highest modularity value of 0.8456 for 22 HSAs when the resolution value is set at 1.38, slightly higher than the highest modularity value of 0.8443 for the 18 ScLeiden-derived HSAs when the resolution value is set at 0.88. In contrast, the ScLouvain method yields 136 HSAs with a modularity of 0.510 when the resolution value is set at 30.23, lower than 0.519 from the 136 ScLeiden-derived HSAs with a resolution value of 29.64. The 136 HSAs derived here are comparable to the 136 Dartmouth HSAs derived in Chapter 4. In addition, the spatial constraints also affect the configuration of HSAs. Readers can refer to C Wang et al. (2021a) for detail.

We also observe similar patterns from the 1,500 scenarios of HRRs for the two methods. Given that a higher modularity value suggests a robust and reliable delineation, the advantage in one method over the other is minor and fluctuates across the scales.

Figure 6.7c shows that the overall computational time[8] generally increases with the number of HSAs by the ScLouvain and ScLeiden methods, especially after the number of HSAs exceeds 10. The minimal computational

---

[7] On an Intel® Xeon® Gold 6140 CPU @ 2.30 GHz 2.29 GHz desktop with a memory of 128GB, it took 9.36 hours for the 1,000 simulations of HSAs and 10.62 hours for the 1,500 simulations of HRRs.

[8] The overall computational time includes reading all data, delineating HSAs by the network community detection method, dissolving HSAs, and calculating several indices.

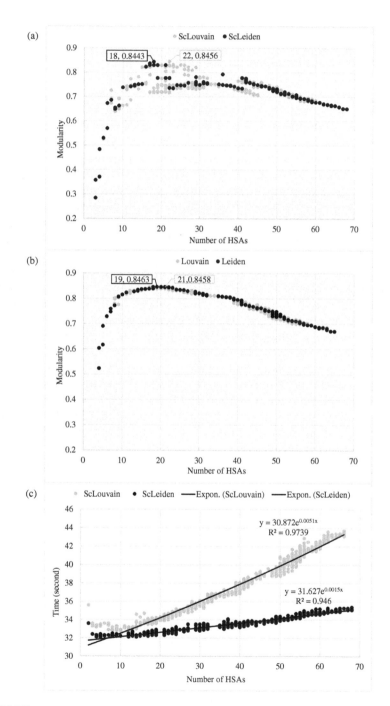

FIGURE 6.7

Modularity versus the number of HSAs for (a) ScLouvain and ScLeiden, and (b) Louvain and Leiden; and (c) computational time versus the number of HSAs for ScLouvain and ScLeiden.

times are 32.8 and 32.1 seconds by the ScLouvain and ScLeiden methods, respectively. Both follow an exponential trend, and the time by the ScLouvain method increases faster than by the ScLeiden method as the number of HSAs increases. On average, the ScLeiden method takes 34 seconds, less than the average of 38 seconds with the ScLouvain method. This is consistent with the finding by Traag et al. (2019) that the Leiden algorithm is slightly faster than the Louvain algorithm.

6.4 Comparing HSAs and HRRs by ScLouvain, ScLeiden, and Refined Dartmouth Methods

Three indices introduced in Chapter 4, namely LI, balanced region size (population), and geographic compactness, are used to evaluate the performance of the methods. Other indices, such as the number of destination ZIP code areas and average travel time, are also presented for information. To be comparable to the 136 HSAs derived from the refined Dartmouth method in Chapter 4, the same number of HSAs (136) is derived by the ScLouvain and ScLeiden methods. In addition, we delineate 22 HSAs by the ScLouvain method with the global optimal modularity value and 18 HSAs by the ScLeiden method with the global optimal modularity value. The results are reported in Table 6.1.

We firstly compare the HSAs by the two network community detection methods. As shown in Table 6.1, the two methods yield similar modularity values with a slight edge to the ScLouvain over ScLeiden (0.846 vs. 0.844). The mean LI of the 18 HSAs from the ScLeiden method is higher than that of the 22 HSAs from the ScLouvain method (0.909 vs. 0.869) as fewer and larger HSAs are more likely to contain more intra-HSA flows. The range of LI from the ScLeiden method is significantly narrower than that from the ScLouvain method (0. 727–0.985 vs. 0.286–1) and is consistent with the difference in the standard deviations (0.065 vs. 0.154). Thus, the ScLeiden method is more favorable in capturing local health care markets than the ScLouvain method. The ScLeiden method yields HSAs with a larger average population (1,045,000 vs. 855,000) with less variability (743,000 vs. 765,000) and thus more balanced in region size than the ScLouvain method. The HSAs by the ScLeiden method have a higher average PAC value than those by the Louvain method (3.191 vs. 2.927) and thus are less compact. Overall, the ScLeiden method outperforms the ScLouvain method in terms of defining global optimal HSAs with a higher average LI, a narrower range of LI values, and more balanced region size, though less compact in shape. Such advantages are more obvious when comparing the same number (136) of HSAs derived from two methods. The ScLeiden method yields HSAs with the same average LI value (0.472) and more balanced population sizes (77,000 vs 80,000 in standard deviation), but slightly less compact in shape (2.181 vs. 2.179 in average PAC) than the ScLouvain method.

TABLE 6.1

Indices for various HSAs in Florida

		22 HSAs by ScLouvain	18 HSAs by ScLeiden	136 HSAs by ScLouvain	136 HSAs by ScLeiden	136 HSAs by Refined Dartmouth
Resolution		1.38	0.88	30.23	29.64	–
Modularity		0.846	0.844	0.510	0.519	–
No. of	Total	208	208	208	208	208
destination	Mean	9	12	2	2	2
ZIP code	Min	1	2	1	1	1
areas	Max	28	29	5	5	7
	S.D.	7	6	1	1	1
Localization	Mean	0.869	0.909	0.472	0.472	0.513
index (LI)	Min	0.286	0.727	0.001	0.001	0.188
	Max	1	0.985	1	1	1
	S.D.	0.154	0.065	0.228	0.227	0.153
Population	Mean	855	1,045	138	138	138
(in 1,000)	Min	8	53	7	12	6
	Max	3,209	3,234	400	394	602
	S.D.	765	743	80	77	121
Geographic	Mean	2.927	3.191	2.179	2.181	2.200
compactness	Min	1.496	1.731	1.267	1.267	1.267
(PAC)	Max	6.363	6.363	6.071	7.251	7.258
	S.D.	1.204	1.189	0.689	0.743	0.771
Average	Mean	25.022	22.785	20.089	19.961	21.734
travel time	Min	5.325	11.650	5.135	5.135	5.3251
(min)	Max	69.111	64.925	87.763	67.072	91.996
	S.D.	15.868	12.030	12.562	11.432	12.77

Figure 6.8a and b shows the variations of LI across 22 ScLouvain HSAs and 18 ScLeiden HSAs overlaid with hospitalization flows, respectively. In both cases, the boundaries of HSAs align well with the major service flows and demonstrate their scientific soundness. Most of the HSAs (19 out of 22 ScLouvain HSAs and 17 out of 18 ScLeiden HSAs) have their LI values above 0.8. The HSAs by the two methods are also largely consistent, with some discrepancies highlighted in the insets of Figure 6.8c. In the first-row inset, three smaller HSAs with LI values between 0.67 and 1 by the ScLouvain method[9] are merged to form one larger ScLeiden HSA with LI=0.85, and the ScLouvain HSA in the southwest corner becomes a smaller ScLeiden HSA but with a slightly improved LI (0.92 vs. 0.91). The two ScLeiden HSAs are more balanced in region size (696,599–901,405) than the four ScLouvain HSAs (14,158–575,833). In the second-row inset, the lowest LI=0.29 is located

---

[9] A very small Louvain HSA with LI=1 is in dark shade in the middle.

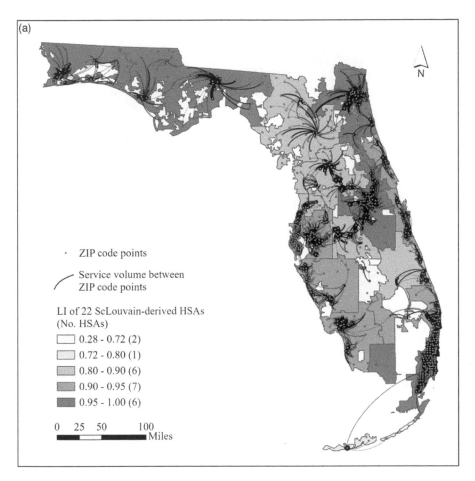

FIGURE 6.8

(a) LI of 22 ScLouvain-derived HSAs with overlaid major service flows (volume ≥150); and (b) LI of 18 ScLeiden-derived HSAs with overlaid major service flows (volume ≥150); and (c) 22 HSAs with ScLouvain versus 18 HSAs with ScLeiden.

(Continued)

at Tavernier, Islamorada, by the ScLouvain method whereas the ScLeiden method has the lowest LI=0.73 in the south. The three ScLeiden HSAs have more balanced region sizes (52,751–3,233,600) than the four ScLouvain HSAs (8,379–3,209,318).

See Appendix B for a user guide on how to use Gephi to create curved-line network flow maps like Figure 6.8a and b.

We now extend the comparison between the 136 HSAs derived by the two methods to the 136 HSAs by the refined Dartmouth method (Table 6.1). The ScLouvain and ScLeiden HSAs enjoy advantages over the refined Dartmouth HSAs in more balanced region size (standard deviation of population size=80,000 and 77,000 versus 121,000) and more compact shape (mean value

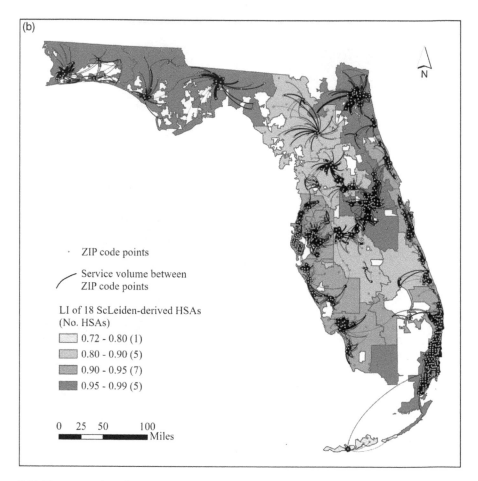

FIGURE 6.8 (*Continued*)
(a) LI of 22 ScLouvain-derived HSAs with overlaid major service flows (volume ≥150); and (b) LI of 18 ScLeiden-derived HSAs with overlaid major service flows (volume ≥150); and (c) 22 HSAs with ScLouvain versus 18 HSAs with ScLeiden.

(Continued)

of PAC=2.179 and 2.181 versus 2.2). However, the refined Dartmouth HSAs have a higher average LI (0.513) than the ScLouvain and ScLeiden HSAs (both 0.472), and their lower bound of LI (0.188) is also significantly higher than those by the two methods (both 0.001). The outlier of an HSA with an extremely low LI = 0.001 by the two network methods is a concern.

The loss of advantage in LI by the two network community detection methods seems to be surprising. We speculate that in the scenario of a large number of HSAs (here 136 HSAs, constructed from 213 destination ZIP code areas), the network community detection methods are not very effective in dividing the network into highly fragmented subnetworks, but their advantages could become more evident when the number of service areas is reduced (e.g., 18–22 HSAs). When the network community detection methods define

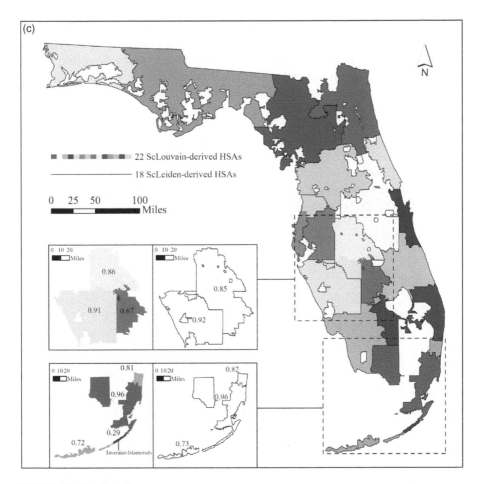

FIGURE 6.8 (Continued)
(a) LI of 22 ScLouvain-derived HSAs with overlaid major service flows (volume ≥150); and (b) LI of 18 ScLeiden-derived HSAs with overlaid major service flows (volume ≥150); and (c) 22 HSAs with ScLouvain versus 18 HSAs with ScLeiden.

the set of HSAs with a global optimal modularity, it suggests that such a configuration captures the organic structure of a health care market where many hospitals have overlapping patient bases and their service areas are tangled together to an inseparable degree. The methods let the structure of a health care market dictate the number of HSAs to be derived, unlike the Dartmouth method that lets the number of hospitals be the primary driver for determining the number of HSAs. Indeed, as revealed in Chapter 4, a significant number of hospitals are too close to each other to have their own HSAs. The overall high LI values in the "global optimal" HSAs by the network community detection methods demonstrate that major advantage, and in the case of ScLeiden method, the narrow variability of LI (0.727–0.985) is even more impressive. Once again, the Dartmouth method (or its refined version in our case) is not scale-flexible and can only generate one set of HSAs. One cannot use the Dartmouth method to derive a given number of HSAs that is comparable to the 22 and 18 HSAs by the two network community detection methods. In other words, we cannot directly verify the advantages of ScLouvain and ScLeiden over the Dartmouth method for delineating smaller numbers of HSAs. More studies need to be conducted to reach a consensus.

Due to the similarity of the 136 HSAs derived by the ScLouvain and ScLeiden methods, hereafter only the result derived from the ScLeiden method is used for comparison. Figure 6.9a and b shows the boundaries of the 136 HSAs derived from the ScLeiden method are largely consistent with the major service flows, while those by the refined Dartmouth method enclose the highest service volumes. The ScLeiden method yields more HSAs

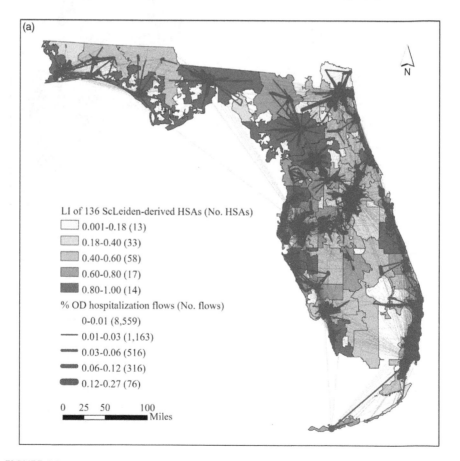

FIGURE 6.9
(a) LI of 136 ScLeiden-derived HSAs with overlaid service flows; (b) LI of 136 Dartmouth comparable HSAs with overlaid service flows; and (c) 136 HSAs with ScLeiden versus those with the refined Dartmouth method.

(Continued)

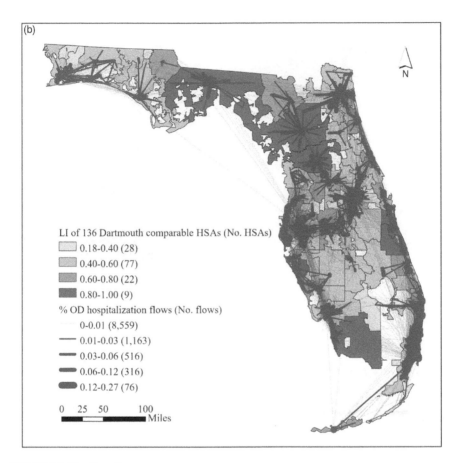

FIGURE 6.9 (Continued)
(a) LI of 136 ScLeiden-derived HSAs with overlaid service flows; (b) LI of 136 Dartmouth comparable HSAs with overlaid service flows; and (c) 136 HSAs with ScLeiden versus those with the refined Dartmouth method.

(Continued)

with $0.18<\text{LI}\leq0.40$ (33) than the refined Dartmouth method (28), but does a better job in delineating HSAs with LI>0.80 (14) than the refined Dartmouth method (9). Both have the most HSAs with LI values between 0.4 and 0.6. Figure 6.9c shows that the boundaries of most HSAs by the ScLeiden and refined Dartmouth methods do not match.

We now present and discuss the results of HRRs. We begin with HRR delineations based on the cardiovascular surgery and neurosurgery flows. The 136 HSAs derived from the ScLouvain and ScLeiden methods are further aggregated to 22 and 20 HRRs with the global optimal modularity, respectively. Similarly, to be comparable to the 59 HRRs derived from the refined Dartmouth method, we have tried to generate the same number of HRRs by the two network community detection methods and are able to obtain

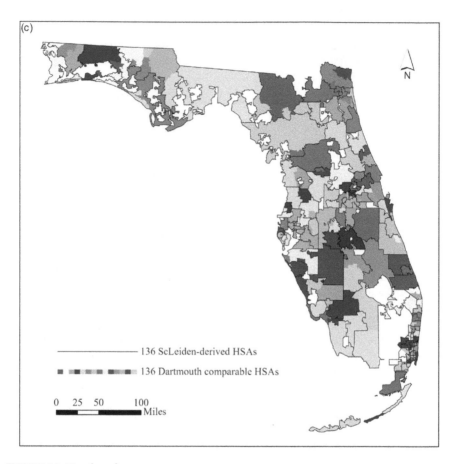

FIGURE 6.9 (*Continued*)
(a) LI of 136 ScLeiden-derived HSAs with overlaid service flows; (b) LI of 136 Dartmouth comparable HSAs with overlaid service flows; and (c) 136 HSAs with ScLeiden versus those with the refined Dartmouth method.

59 HRRs by the ScLouvain method and 58 HRRs by the ScLeiden method[10] (Table 6.2).

Based on the results reported in Table 6.2, the ScLeiden method generates 2 fewer HRRs with the global optimal modularity than the ScLouvain method (20 vs. 22). The 20 ScLeiden HRRs have a higher average modularity value (0.7909 vs. 0.7905) and a higher average LI (0.883 vs. 0.880) and are more balanced in region size (standard deviation=513,000 vs. 577,000), but less

---

[10] We attempted different resolution values, and the ScLeiden method could only derive either 58 or 60 HRRs. Fifty-eight HRRs were selected with a resolution value 11.96, identical to that used for deriving the 59 HRRs derived from the ScLouvain method. This resolution value used by the ScLeiden method also had the highest modularity value among various resolution values for generating the same number (58) of HRRs.

TABLE 6.2

Indices for Various HRRs Based on Cardiovascular Surgery and Neurosurgery Flows in Florida

		22 HRRs by ScLouvain	20 HRRs by ScLeiden	59 HRRs by ScLouvain	58 HRRs by ScLeiden	59 HRRs by Refined Dartmouth
Resolution		1.75	1.75	11.96	11.96	–
Modularity		0.7905	0.7909	0.6487	0.6613	–
Localization index (LI)	Mean	0.880	0.883	0.669	0.681	0.654
	Min	0.721	0.729	0.041	0.150	0.310
	Max	0.984	0.984	0.971	0.971	0.971
	S.D.	0.069	0.072	0.187	0.162	0.167
Population (in 1,000)	Mean	855	940	319	324	319
	Min	157	157	125	125	124
	Max	2,509	2,124	1,043	852	974
	S.D.	577	513	163	149	185
Geographic compactness (PAC)	Mean	2.928	2.945	2.410	2.401	2.399
	Min	1.570	1.570	1.308	1.308	1.308
	Max	5.379	6.363	5.498	5.513	5.526
	S.D.	1.225	1.351	0.897	0.883	0.933

compact in shape (2.945 vs. 2.928 in PAC) than the 22 HRRs by the ScLouvain method. These differences are minor. As shown in Figure 6.10a and b, the boundaries of HRRs derived from the two methods are well aligned with the interconnected service volumes of cardiovascular surgery and neurosurgery flows between HSAs. Many HRRs are consistent with each other in Figure 6.10c with minor difference in the two insets. The first-row inset shows the ScLeiden method derives one HRR with LI=0.96, while the ScLouvain method generates two HRRs with LI =0.92 and 0.95. In the second-row inset, two HRRs with LI = 0.75 and 0.94 by the ScLeiden are reconfigured to three HRRs with LI = 0.81, 0.90, and 0.76 by the ScLouvain.

The comparison between the 59 ScLouvain HRRs and 58 ScLeiden HRRs from the two methods leads to similar conclusions. The advantages of the ScLeiden method over the ScLouvain method are more evident in their corresponding HRRs: higher average modularity (0.6613 vs. 0.6487), higher average LI (0.681 vs. 0.669), more balanced region size (standard deviation=149,000 vs. 163,000), and being more compact (average PAC=2.401 vs. 2.410). The lower bound of LI by the ScLeiden method is also significantly higher than the lower bound of LI by the ScLouvain method (0.15 vs. 0.041) and thus less variability in standard deviation of LI (0.162 vs. 0.187). With comparison to the 59 Dartmouth HRRs, the HRRs by the two methods have higher mean LI values (0.669 and 0.681 vs. 0.654) and are more balanced in region size (163,000 and 149,000 vs. 185,000), but less compact in shape (2.410 and 2.401 vs. 2.399). Once again, the outlier of an HRR with a low LI value

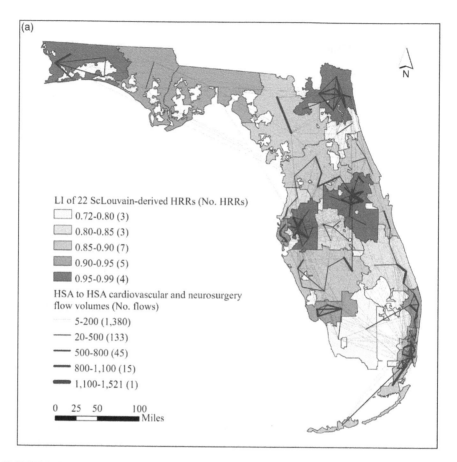

(a)

LI of 22 ScLouvain-derived HRRs (No. HRRs)

　0.72-0.80 (3)
　0.80-0.85 (3)
　0.85-0.90 (7)
　0.90-0.95 (5)
　0.95-0.99 (4)

HSA to HSA cardiovascular and neurosurgery flow volumes (No. flows)

　5-200 (1,380)
　20-500 (133)
　500-800 (45)
　800-1,100 (15)
　1,100-1,521 (1)

0　25　50　　　100
　　　　　　　　　Miles

FIGURE 6.10
(a) LI of 22 ScLouvain-derived HRRs with overlaid service flows; (b) LI of 20 ScLeiden-derived HRRs with overlaid service flows; and (c) 22 HRRs with ScLouvain versus 20 HRRs with ScLeiden.

(Continued)

(0.041 in one of 59 HRRs by the ScLouvain and 0.150 in one of the 58 HRRs by the ScLeiden) is a concern.

As discussed in Chapter 4, one may explore the scenario of using the neurosurgery flows to construct the HRRs. The ScLouvain and ScLeiden methods yield 19 and 18 global optimal HRRs, and 48 Dartmouth comparable HRRs. The results are reported in Table 6.3. Findings are very similar to those based on Table 6.2 and related discussions are omitted here.

To recap, the ScLeiden method is more advantageous than the ScLouvain method for delineating HSAs and HRRs in terms of achieving higher modularity with more computational efficiency, more favorable localization index for capturing the local health care markets of general and tertiary hospitals, and more balanced region size. Their overall advantages over the refined Dartmouth method are more evident when the numbers of HSAs and HRRs become smaller.

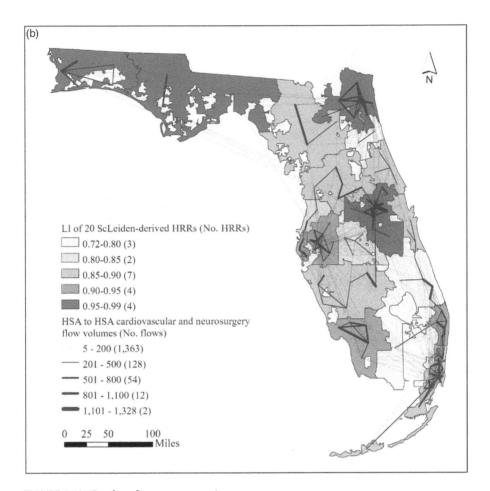

FIGURE 6.10 (*Continued*)
(a) LI of 22 ScLouvain-derived HRRs with overlaid service flows; (b) LI of 20 ScLeiden-derived HRRs with overlaid service flows; and (c) 22 HRRs with ScLouvain versus 20 HRRs with ScLeiden.

(*Continued*)

Another important finding is that the numbers of HSAs and HRRs with the global optimal modularity are close to each other (22 HSAs vs. 22 HRRs; 18 HSAs vs. 20 HRRs) for the two network community detection methods and are far fewer than 136 HSAs and 59 HRRs derived from the refined Dartmouth method. As the numbers of HSAs and HRRs decline, the mean values of LI increase significantly, so do the modularity values increase. This suggests the need of further consolidation of HSAs and HRRs in order to capture the general and tertiary hospital markets that both are increasingly integrated and interwoven. The numbers of HSAs and HRRs by the refined Dartmouth methods might be too high. Once again, more work is needed to determine the most appropriate choice about the numbers of HSAs and HRRs.

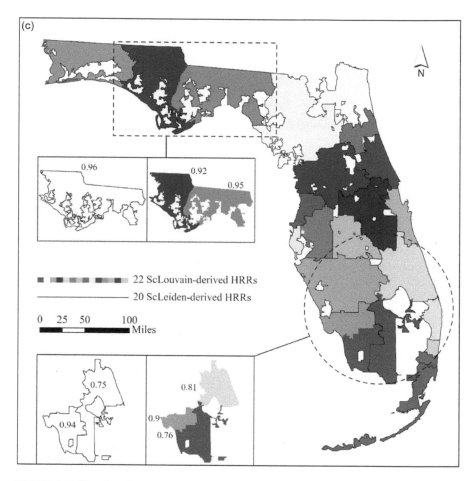

FIGURE 6.10 (*Continued*)
(a) LI of 22 ScLouvain-derived HRRs with overlaid service flows; (b) LI of 20 ScLeiden-derived HRRs with overlaid service flows; and (c) 22 HRRs with ScLouvain versus 20 HRRs with ScLeiden.

6.5 Summary

This chapter introduced the network community detection approach to define HSAs by grouping most densely interconnected areas into HSAs while keeping apart the least connected areas. In comparison with the Dartmouth method and the Huff model that rely on the plurality rule, this approach has a systematic perspective to pursue the maximum connections within derived HSAs.

The network community detection approach is built upon a rich body of community detection algorithms in the complex network science literature.

TABLE 6.3

Indices for Various HRRs Based on Neurosurgery Flows in Florida

		19 HRRs by ScLouvain	18 HRRs by ScLeiden	48 HRRs by ScLouvain	48 HRRs by ScLeiden	48 HRRs by Refined Dartmouth
Resolution		2.33	2.13	8.87	8.84	−
Modularity		0.7381	0.7358	0.5567	0.5766	−
Localization index (LI)	Mean	0.818	0.820	0.580	0.581	0.567
	Min	0.600	0.595	0.031	0.151	0.223
	Max	0.982	0.982	0.923	0.923	0.984
	S.D.	0.102	0.109	0.198	0.182	0.202
Population (in 1,000)	Mean	990	1,045	400	392	392
	Min	345	462	125	125	125
	Max	2,281	2,201	915	852	1,240
	S.D.	555	518	176	167	267
Geographic compactness (PAC)	Mean	2.989	3.023	2.522	2.535	2.513
	Min	1.530	1.570	1.425	1.520	1.314
	Max	6.363	6.363	5.546	5.546	6.523
	S.D.	1.322	1.342	0.944	0.918	1.073

This chapter covers two methods, namely the popular Louvain algorithm and the more recent Leiden algorithm. The latter is proposed specifically to rectify some of the deficiencies in the former, such as poorly connected or disconnected communities. Guided by maximizing a quality measure such as modularity, the Louvain and Leiden methods generate a series of communities corresponding to various resolutions and thus are scale-flexible. In other words, users can derive a certain number of communities by adjusting the resolution value. Adopting the Louvain and Leiden algorithms for delineating HSAs needs to account for some spatial constraints such as spatial contiguity and, in the case of HRRs, a threshold population size. Such methods are therefore termed "spatially constrained Louvain (ScLouvain)" and "spatially constrained Leiden (ScLeiden)" methods. The originals are referred to as "aspatial Louvain method" and "aspatial Leiden method".

Automated tools are developed to implement the ScLouvain and ScLeiden methods as well as their aspatial counterparts. All are highly computationally efficient, and in our case study, the delineation of HSAs in Florida takes less than a minute. As the number of HSAs increases, the computational time increases. The ScLouvain method takes slightly more time than the ScLeiden method. The ScLeiden method generally yields more favorable HSAs with a higher average LI and more balanced region size than the ScLouvain method. In comparison with the refined Dartmouth method implemented in Chapter 4, the advantages of the two network community detection methods become more evident in delineating fewer HSAs. In other words, when the number of HSAs is close to the number of ZIP code areas with hospitals, the Dartmouth method is efficient and effective to delineate local health care markets that are limited in spatial range, but when it is needed to derive a smaller number (e.g., the global optimal number) of HSAs that truly captures the interwoven network structure, the two network community detection methods show significant advantages. Moreover, the Dartmouth method only yields one set (i.e., a fixed number) of HSAs whereas the network community detection methods derive a series of HSAs with various resolutions and suggests what number of HSAs be the optimal delineation.

7

Delineating Cancer Service Areas in the Northeast Region of the USA

This chapter discusses the application of delineation of service areas for a specialized health care, cancer care. Cancer is the second leading cause of death in the USA. Cancer care is identified as a distinct patient population with unique sets of services, needs, technologies, and clinical specializations. Innovations in oncology care, complex treatment paradigms, and specialty settings are likely to create distinct health care markets from hospital service areas (HSAs) for cancer patients (IOM, 2014). The choice of spatial units with which to measure disease and related care and outcomes is important for appropriately assessing how well cancer incidence, prevalence, and survival are aligned with the resources needed to address those. A new system of cancer service areas (CSAs) is needed to best evaluate cancer care utilization, assess cancer-centered outcomes, identify actionable disparities, and optimize resource allocation.

A case study of delineating CSAs in the Northeast Region of the USA is used to demonstrate how CSAs may differ from the general HSAs, and thus the need of defining health service areas pertaining to specific service types, as advocated in Chapter 1. Given the complexity and constant advancement of medical treatments, there is a rich set of health cares classified into various specializations. There is also the need for defining service areas that vary in geographic scope and scale and temporally. It highlights the value of developing automated, user-friendly, and efficient methods. The methods illustrated in Chapters 4–6 meet this challenge. The assessment in Section 6.4 of Chapter 6 suggests that when data are available, the network community detection approach, specifically the ScLouvain and ScLeiden methods, be the most promising choice. The case study offers us an opportunity to illustrate how the methods and skills learned from the previous chapters are utilized together in defining a distinctive type of health care service areas.

Based on our recent work reported in multiple papers (F Wang et al., 2020; C Wang et al., 2021a, b), this chapter focuses on highlighting the uniqueness of CSAs. Section 7.1 outlines the data sources for the case study. Section 7.2 introduces a method of interpolating data of suppressed service flows in preparation of network analysis. Section 7.3 discusses the results of delineated CSAs and highlights the difference from the Dartmouth HRRs. Section 7.4 explores how the distance decay behavior in cancer care patients varies across the CSAs. Section 7.5 concludes the chapter with a summary.

DOI: 10.1201/9780429260285-7

7.1 Study Area and Cancer Care Data

The study area is the nine-state Northeast Census Region (Maine, New Hampshire, Vermont, Massachusetts, Connecticut, Rhode Island, New York, New Jersey, and Pennsylvania) in the USA, hereafter referred to as "Northeast Region" (Figure 7.1).

Data for patients were extracted from the Medicare beneficiary denominator file from the Centers for Medicare and Medicaid Services (CMS). Patients were enrolled in Medicare Parts A and B, aged 65–99 years, from January 1, 2014, to September 30, 2015. Cancer patients were identified using diagnosis codes listed for 26 cancer types (NCI, 2014). Cancer services included cancer-directed surgical procedures, chemotherapy, and radiation treatment codes.

The spatial data included both the polygon and point layers of ZIP code areas, and the latter was the population-weighted centroids of ZIP code areas, calibrated from the 2010 census population data at the census block level. Point ZIP codes (typically associated with large business entities) were aggregated to the ZIP code areas that enclosed those points. Service volumes were calculated for each origin–destination (OD) ZIP code pair, where the

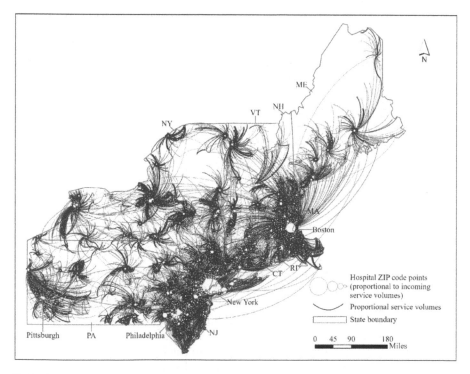

FIGURE 7.1
Network of cancer service volumes between ZIP code areas in Northeast USA (2014–2015).

origin was the patient ZIP code of residence and the destination was the ZIP code of provider(s). Per CMS data use agreement, volumes of less than 11 were suppressed and needed to be interpolated as illustrated in Section 7.2. Since both patient residence and hospitals were geocoded to ZIP code areas, the network of patient service volumes was constructed between ZIP code areas.

Another important data preparation task for the case study was to estimate drive time between ZIP code areas in the study area. That was accomplished by a differential sampling approach as illustrated in Section 2.5 of Chapter 2. In short, as trip lengths increased, we used simpler methods that utilized less data with shorter computational time to derive preliminary estimates of drive time. We only used a more accurate method (i.e., via the Google Maps API) to estimate a small fraction of the OD trips by random sampling, derived a set of empirical models on the relationship between preliminary lower-computational-cost estimates and the more accurate estimates, and adjusted the preliminary estimates accordingly. The sampling intensity dropped for long-range trips as the desirability for precision of drive time estimates also declined, and thus saved computational time without much compromise in quality of the results.

For the study area, the network contains 5,969 nodes (represented by the ZIP code centroids) and 86,192 edges (i.e., service flows between ZIP code areas) with the total service volumes (sum of edge weights) of 2,443,538. As shown in Figure 7.1, the network is composed of nodes and edges linking the nodes, and here the circle size represents the total service volume ending at a node (ZIP code area), and the thickness of a flow line reflects the service volume between two nodes. Note that the service volumes included both directions between two ZIP code areas and thus the network is undirected. Large cities such as New York, Boston, and Philadelphia anchored major destinations for cancer services in the region with interwoven complex service flows, and the rest of the region was served by smaller local hospitals drawing patients from their surrounding areas.

7.2 Interpolating Suppressed Service Volumes

As stated previously, service volumes between ZIP code areas with values smaller than 11 were suppressed. Among the total of $n = 86,192$ edges with non-zero service volumes, 56,317 OD pairs (about two-third, 65.3% to be precise) have their service volumes suppressed. A network without the suppressed service volumes would be highly fragmented, and analysis based on such a partial network would not yield any meaningful delineation of CSAs. This section illustrates how to interpolate the missing service volumes for the $n_B = 56,317$ OD pairs (subset B) from the $n_A = 29,875$ observed service volumes on corresponding OD pairs (subset A) by three steps. Data suppression for small population samples to protect patients' geoprivacy is a common challenge for health data analysts (Mu et al., 2015). The technique discussed here may benefit analysts with similar challenges.

First, a gravity-based regression model is used to fit the observed service volumes between ZIP code areas from data subset A.

Recall the gravity model in Equation 3.1 in Sub-section 3.3.1 of Chapter 3. It is refined as

$$T_{ij} = a\left(O_i D_j\right)^\alpha f\left(d_{ij}\right) \tag{7.1}$$

where T_{ij} is the number of service volumes from ZIP code area i to ZIP code area j, O_i and D_j are the total service volumes originated from i and ending at j, respectively, d_{ij} is the travel time between them, a is a scalar, α is the elasticity parameter for the product term $(O_i D_j)$ (assuming an identical elasticity for O_i and D_j), and f is a function of travel time d_{ij}. Instead of assuming a unitary elasticity $(\alpha=1)$ in Equation 3.1, here we add an elasticity parameter α to the term $(O_i D_j)$. Permitting the variability of α adds one more explanatory variable in fitting the gravity model and improves the fitting power.

As illustrated in Sub-section 3.3.1, different distance decay functions are tested in corresponding regressions on data subset A (n_A=29,875), and the best-fitting model is identified. The popular power function (in its log-transformation) yields the highest R^2=0.234, and the result is

$$\ln T_{ij} = 2.0361 + 0.2445 \ln\left(O_i D_j\right) - 0.4309 \ln d_{ij} \tag{7.2}$$

The second step uses the derived gravity model in Equation 7.2 to obtain the preliminary estimator $\hat{T}_{ij}$ for service volumes based on data subset B.

In the data acquisition process, we were able to obtain the product value of $O_i D_j$ from the CMS, with the same threshold value of 11 applied. In the study area, only a negligible number (n_{B2}=15) of records in the study area had the values of $O_i D_j$ less than 11 and were suppressed, and none in subset A and all in subset B. The vast majority of subset B, n_{B1}=56,317−15=56,302, had valid values of $O_i D_j$. Plugging the values of $O_i D_j$ and d_{ij} from this part of data subset B1 into Equation 7.2 and solving for T_{ij} yield the preliminary estimated service volumes, denoted as $\hat{T}_{ij}$. Its values range from 3 to 107.

The final step is to further adjust the preliminary estimator $\hat{T}_{ij}$ to $\hat{T}'_{ij}$ so that its values fall within its feasible range [1,10]. For the part of data subset n_{B1}=56,302, a simple monotonic transformation $\hat{T}'_{ij} = 2 \ln \hat{T}_{ij}$ serves the purpose, and its values are rounded to integers. In other words,

$$\hat{T}'_{ij} = 2 \ln \hat{T}_{ij} = 2\left(2.0361 + 0.2445 \ln\left(O_i D_j\right) - 0.4309 \ln d_{ij}\right) \tag{7.3}$$

For the other part of data subset with n_{B2}=15 records of suppressed $O_i D_j$ (i.e., the lowest non-zero value), we can simply assume $\hat{T}'_{ij} = 1$.

The rescaling of the preliminary estimator $\hat{T}_{ij}$ to $\hat{T}'_{ij}$ for the lower volume trips recognizes that the distance decay effect in cancer service volumes may be captured by different functions in various travel time ranges. That is to say, the *fitted* distance decay function from observed data to capture higher service volumes $(T_{ij} \geq 11)$ is a power function such as $f(d_{ij}) = c_1 d_{ij}^{-0.4309}$, and its monotonic transform $f(d_{ij}) = c_2 - 0.8618 \ln d_{ij}$ (i.e., a logarithmic function) is assumed as the new distance decay function for interpolating suppressed lower service volumes $\hat{T}'_{ij}$ so that $\hat{T}'_{ij} \in [1,10]$. Figure 7.2 shows how the two distance decay functions differ.

In summary, the final complete set of 86,192 records of service volumes that define the edge weights between ZIP code areas i and j in the network is composed of

1. the subset A $(n_A=29{,}875)$ with observed $T_{ij} \geq 11$ and observed O_iD_j, based on which the regression model in Equation 7.2 is derived;
2. the subset B1 $(n_{B1}=56{,}302)$ with suppressed T_{ij} and observed $O_iD_j \geq 11$, now updated with interpolated $\hat{T}'_{ij}$ based on Equation 7.3, where $\hat{T}'_{ij} \in [1,10]$; and
3. the subset B2 $(n_{B2}=15)$ with suppressed T_{ij} and suppressed O_iD_j, now updated with interpolated $\hat{T}'_{ij} = 1$.

The whole process is summarized in a flow chart in Figure 7.3.

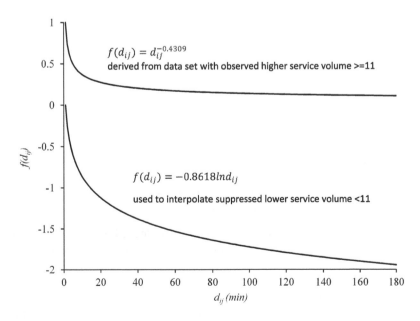

FIGURE 7.2
Distance decay functions for higher and lower service volumes.

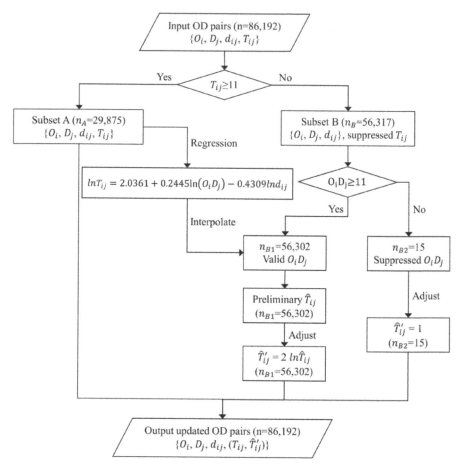

FIGURE 7.3
Workflow of interpolating suppressed OD service volumes.

7.3 Delineating CSAs by ScLouvain and ScLeiden in the Northeast Region

This case study adopts the network community detection approach, namely the ScLouvain and ScLeiden methods, for delineating the CSAs in the Northeast Region of the USA. Chapter 6 discussed the technical details of both methods, and this section focuses on practical issues unique to the CSAs in the study area.

Several rules are implemented to ensure spatial adjacency and minimum region size of the derived CSAs:

1. *The spatial adjacency rule.* Both the ScLouvain and ScLeiden methods apply their corresponding aspatial community detection algorithms initially and generate communities that may be spatially non-contiguous. Each of these non-contiguous communities is split into multiple sub-communities, each of which forms a contiguous polygon and thus a new node in the network. The spatial network is updated with the new nodes and new edges.

2. *The geographic island rule.* The study area has some ZIP code areas off the east coast. They are geographic islands, but connect with the mainland via ferryboats, bridges, or other means with non-zero service volumes. To fully incorporate these areas in the CSA delineation, a virtual bridge is constructed between an island (composed of one or multiple ZIP code areas) and its nearest ZIP code area on the mainland. Such a virtual bridge is represented as a link in the spatial adjacency matrix.

3. *The orphan node rule.* "An orphan node" refers to a node (ZIP code area or an intermediate community in the process) with no edges (zero service volume) linking to any other units. An orphan node is merged to its neighboring node with the smallest population size to help balance region size for derived CSAs, a desirable property in regionalization, without compromising the overall modularity.

4. *The threshold size rule.* The Dartmouth HRRs used a population of 120,000 as the threshold size. Similarly, cancer care is a highly specialized health care, and the same threshold of 120,000 is imposed on the delineation of CSAs. Any intermediate small community is merged to its neighbor to attain positive modularity gain till the threshold size is reached.

Enforcing the above four rules has substantial impacts on increasing computational time and reducing modularity. Given the efficiency of both algorithms, the increased computational times remain very reasonable after imposing the constraints.[1] Understandably, the modularity decreases at the cost of splitting up those enclaved or enclosed communities to ensure spatial continuity.

As stated in Chapter 6, the two methods are scale-flexible and can generate a series of different numbers of CSAs corresponding to user-defined resolutions. Here only the scenario of 43 CSAs is selected for evaluation, which is comparable to 43 Dartmouth HRRs in the study area. Table 7.1 shows

---

[1] For our case study on the network of 5,969 nodes and 89,162 service flows, the computational time ranged from 5 to 150 seconds as the number of CSAs converged from 70 to 1 in a desktop of Inter(R) Core(TM) i7-4770 CPU@ 3.40 GHz with 32 GB of memory. The ScLeiden method was slightly more efficient with less computational time than the ScLouvain method.

TABLE 7.1

Basic Statistics of Indices for Various CSAs and HRRs in the Northeast Region

Method		43 CSAs		43 HRRs
		ScLeiden	ScLouvain	Dartmouth
Modularity		0.601	0.597	0.698
Localization index (LI)	Min	0.407	0.411	0.185
	Max	0.974	0.974	0.967
	Mean	0.746	0.745	0.676
	S.D.	0.145	0.145	0.178
Geographic compactness	Min	1.560	1.560	1.536
(PAC)	Max	7.379	7.379	7.834
	Mean	3.056	3.054	3.138
	S.D.	1.021	1.051	1.535
Balance in region size	Min	159	159	200
(population in 1,000)	Max	4,328	4,300	4,815
	Mean	1,270	1,270	1,265
	S.D.	987	993	1,213

Note: S.D. stands for standard deviation.

the statistics for three indices, namely localization index (LI), compactness, and balance in region size, by the two methods (ScLouvain and ScLeiden) in comparison with the original Dartmouth HRRs. See Sub-section 4.4.2 of Chapter 4 for descriptions of the three indices.

Between the two network community detection methods, the ScLeiden method yields CSAs with a slightly higher average LI (0.746 vs. 0.745) and more balanced region size (standard deviation=987,000 vs. 993,000) than the ScLouvain method, but slightly less compact in shape (average PAC=3.056 vs. 3.054). Overall, the ScLeiden method outperforms the ScLouvain method in higher LIs and more balanced region size in derived CSAs. With comparison to the 43 Dartmouth HRRs, the advantages are far more obvious for the CSAs by the two methods: The mean LI values are 0.746 and 0.745 for the CSAs vs. 0.676 for the HRRs, the mean PAC is 3.056 and 3.054 for the CSAs vs. 3.138 for the HRRs, and the standard deviations of population sizes are 987,000 and 993,000 for the CSAs vs. 1,213,000 for the HRRs. Both the ScLouvain and ScLeiden methods optimize the network segmentation with a clear objective of maximizing modularity and yield notably high LIs. Their advantages over the Dartmouth method are clear. The derived CSAs enjoy higher LIs, more compact shape, and more balanced region size than their Dartmouth HRR counterparts.

This once again demonstrates the values of deriving a distinctive service area unit for cancer care instead of simply adopting the generic HRRs to capture the cancer care market structure. Between the two network community detection methods, the comparative advantage of ScLeiden over ScLouvain in average LI value and computational time is evident. A high LI value is considered the most important objective in HSA delineation. Even a minor improvement in LI by the Leiden algorithm over a widely popular Louvain algorithm (and here their spatial counterparts), considered revolutionary at the time of its conception, is not an easy feat.

Figure 7.4 shows 43 ScLeiden-derived CSAs overlaid with the service flows. Each CSA encloses major service flows of cancer patients while flows between CSAs appear negligible. The map obtained by overlaying the 43 ScLouvain-derived CSAs and the service flows reveals a similar pattern and is not shown here. That is to say, both ScLouvain and ScLeiden capture cancer care markets composed of tightly connected ZIP code areas via service volumes. As shown in Figure 7.5, the ScLeiden and ScLouvain methods derive CSAs with largely consistent boundaries with some minor discrepancies. The upper-left inset shows that both the methods divide the area into three CSAs, but with different spatial configurations. While the LIs differ little between the two (average LI=0.877 for the three ScLeiden-derived CSAs on the right side, slightly lower than the average LI=0.880 for the three ScLouvain-derived CSAs on the left side), the ScLeiden method seems to yield more balanced region size among the three CSAs than the ScLouvain (by

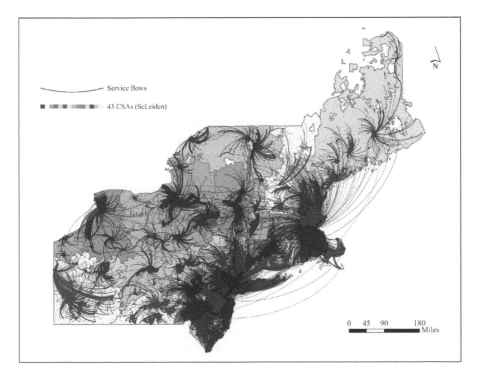

FIGURE 7.4
43 ScLeiden-derived CSAs vs. service flows.

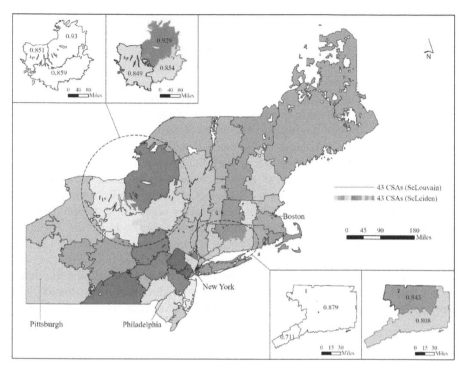

FIGURE 7.5
ScLouvain-derived vs. ScLeiden-derived CSAs.

expanding the smallest CSA southward). The lower-right inset shows how the ScLouvain and ScLeiden methods segment the area into two CSAs differently. The ScLeiden method yields two CSAs with more similar LIs (0.843 and 0.808) than the ScLouvain method (0.879 and 0.711), and the improvement of LI in one (0.808−0.711=0.097) clearly offsets more than the loss of LI in another (0.879−0.843=0.036). Once again, the ScLeiden method outperforms the ScLouvain method in deriving CSAs that are better connected and more balanced in population size.

Figure 7.6 overlays the 43 Dartmouth HRRs with the service flows and reveals that the HRRs are less well suited to capture the cancer care market. Due to the similarity between the two sets of derived CSAs, only the 43 ScLeiden-derived CSAs are overlaid with the same number of HRRs, as shown in Figure 7.7. The discrepancies are apparent, and the advantages of CSAs derived by the ScLeiden method are evident over the Dartmouth HRRs. Here two areas are highlighted as examples to illustrate the gaps. The upper-left inset in Figure 7.7 shows that the CSAs at the south corner (Pittsburgh region) with highly interwoven service flows, and the CSA with a high LI of 0.974 is split into three HRRs with much lower LIs, indicating an expanded coverage of cancer-related services that attract more people from distant places. The lower-right inset in Figure 7.7 shows that four CSAs

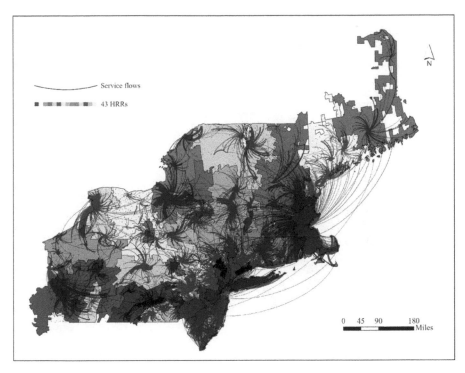

FIGURE 7.6
43 HRRs vs. service flows.

with relatively high LIs in the Boston area are contained in one mega-HRR. Decomposition of such a large HRR is favorable because it helps balance the CSA size and enables researchers to measure possible variations within it.

7.4 Variation of Distance Decay Behavior across CSAs in the Northeast Region

Following the case study presented in Section 7.3, this section examines the variability of spatial behavior in distance decay for cancer care utilization across geographic areas in the same study area, Northeast Region of the USA. Sub-section 3.3.2 of Chapter 3 examines the variation of distance decay behavior of hospitalization across different types of geographic areas such as income levels or urbanicities of individual patient's residence. Here, the variation is across contiguous geographic areas over space. As stated earlier in this chapter, the analysis unit used in a study needs to pertain to the service type under examination (here, cancer care) and reflects the market area of that service (here, the very CSAs derived). The distance decay behavior

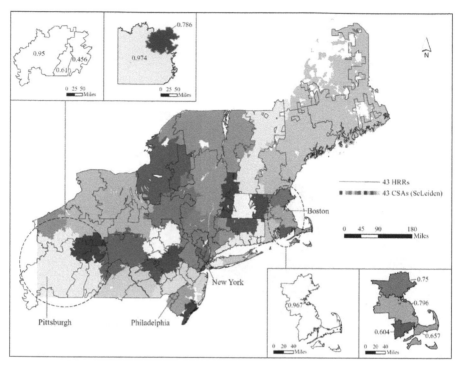

FIGURE 7.7
43 ScLeiden-derived CSAs vs. 43 HRRs.

can be measured by a simple average travel time for patients in an area, or by the distance friction coefficient in a continuous function. Most studies in the literature use the former, and few employ the latter approach. The classic study on the spatial variability of distance decay coefficient was conducted by Fotheringham (1981), which found that the distance friction was weaker in better developed regions with better-connected road networks. Here, both average travel time and distance decay coefficient are used.

For the overall service volumes in the Northeast Region, 46.8% travelled less than 30 minutes, 85.5% travelled within 60 minutes, and 99.6% travelled within 180 minutes to seek cancer care by automobile driving. The travel times had the mean value of 46.97 minutes and median value of 37.23 minutes. Given the small proportion of service volume beyond 180 minutes (0.4%), we cap the travel time at 180 minutes in the distance decay analysis. Figure 7.8a plots the percentage and cumulative percentage of service volume on travel time (bandwidth=2 minutes). The distribution peaks at 25 minutes. A minor peak at 5 minutes is attributable to the dominance (97.9%) of intra-zonal travel time (proportional to ZIP code area size) for trips within 10 minutes. For those 34% patient visits within 25 minutes, patients may be relatively indifferent (or less sensitive) to increasing travel time for cancer care, and the general upward trend is most likely attributable to the given spatial distribution of cancer care facilities and the aforementioned issue of intra-zonal travel time estimation. Beyond 25 minutes, it exhibits a distinct distance decay effect of patient visits as the travel time increases.

Figure 7.8b shows the *complementary cumulative distribution* of service volumes, as illustrated in Section 3.4 of Chapter 3, which is the approach adopted here for analyzing the distance decay behavior. Following the five

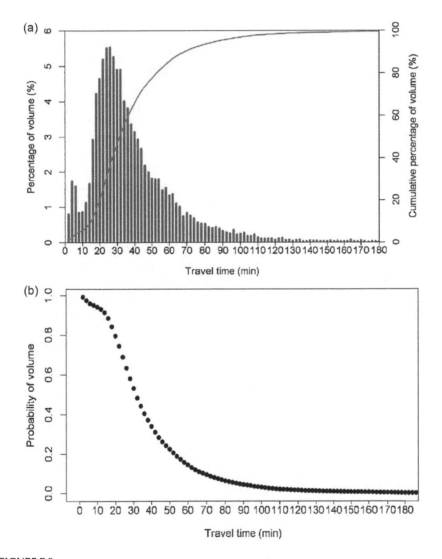

FIGURE 7.8
(a) Percentage and cumulative percentage of service volume vs. travel time, and (b) complementary cumulative distribution of service volume vs. travel time.

TABLE 7.2

Regressions on the Log-Transforms of Five Distance Decay Functions for Cancer Care in the Northeast USA

Distance Decay Function	Function Used in Regression	a	β	R^2
Square-root exponential	$\log I = a - \beta\sqrt{d}$	2.147	0.563	0.974
Exponential	$\log I = a - \beta d$	**0.179**	**0.034**	**0.989**
Normal	$\log I = a - \beta d^2$	−1.027	0.0002	0.888
Power/Pareto	$\log I = a - \beta \log d$	4.494	1.754	0.827
Log-normal	$\log I = a - \beta(\log d)^2$	1.949	0.260	0.937

functions in Table 3.2 of Chapter 3, the linear regression results on their log-transformed models are reported in Table 7.2. The exponential function is the best in fitting the distance decay curve (shown in Figure 7.8b), followed by the square-root exponential, log-normal, normal, and power functions. This is consistent with the finding in Jia et al. (2019) that the exponential function is the best to capture the spatial behaviors of human movements in a singular decay parameter estimation when using the complementary cumulative distribution curve.

The regression analysis on the distance decay effect of service volumes in each of the 43 CSAs shows that the exponential distance decay function enjoys the best-fitting power in most of the CSAs and is highly significant at the 0.001 level in all 43 CSAs. In order to maintain consistency and enable comparison, our discussion focuses on the regression results from the exponential function. Figures 7.9 and 7.10 show the spatial distributions of mean travel time and distance friction coefficient across the 43 CSAs, respectively. In Figure 7.9, the lowest mean travel time is 31 minutes, followed by other four CSAs (three are averaging 33 minutes and one is 34 minutes) in New York City and its adjacent areas. Cancer patients in the CSA to south of Boston (the coastal CSA including the islands) have the longest travel time averaging 72 minutes. In Figure 7.10, two highly urbanized clusters stand out at the top with the highest friction coefficients: 1 CSA in New Jersey with a friction coefficient of 0.064 and 2 CSAs around Boston with a friction coefficient of 0.055. From these two clusters, the distance decay effect gradually declines outward with lower friction coefficients.

Several factors may help us understand the variability of distance decay effect, measured in mean travel time and distance friction coefficient, across the CSAs. Public health also has a long tradition of examining the effect of urbanicity (i.e., degree of urbanization) on health behavior and outcome including cancer (e.g., McLafferty and Wang, 2009). Urbanicity is defined by two variables here: *urbanization ratio* and *density of population over 65*. For each CSA, the urbanization ratio is calculated by the

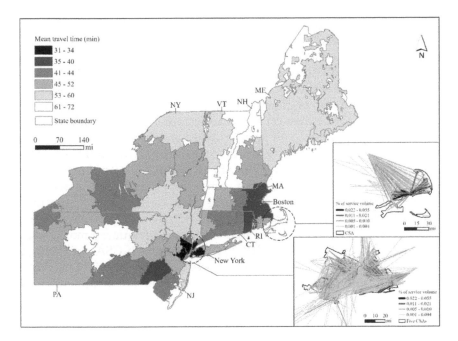

FIGURE 7.9
Mean travel times in the 43 CSAs.

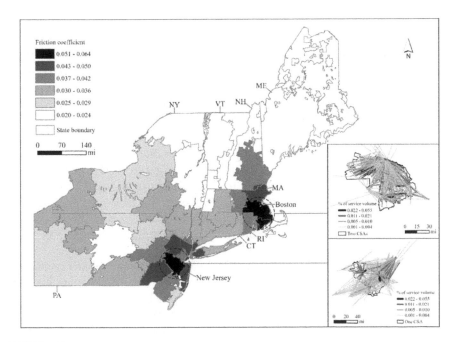

FIGURE 7.10
Distance friction coefficients in the 43 CSAs.

population in urban areas over total population. Here urban areas include both "urbanized areas" and "urban clusters" defined in geographic units of fine scale such as census tract and census block by the US census for better accuracy (Xu and Wang, 2015). Population density (persons per square km) is considered another proxy to capture urbanicity in terms of land use intensity by human settlement, and here we limit population to those over 65 because of our data on Medicare population. Economic development level is also believed to affect travel behavior as better-developed regions tend to have better transportation infrastructure and is measured by *median household income* and *poverty rate for population over 65* in this study. As stated previously, a more competitive health care market may drive or facilitate patients to seek cares afar. Here, market structure is defined by the *Herfindahl–Hirschman Index (HHI)* and LI, commonly used in health studies (Hu et al., 2018). HHI is the sum of squared market share of patient visits in destination ZIP codes within each CSA, and a higher HHI indicates more concentrated (as opposed to competitive) market. LI is the ratio of service volumes within a CSA over the total service volumes originated from the same CSA and measures the degree of local hospitalization.

The correlation matrices for the two distance decay measures (mean travel time "MeanTime" in minutes, and friction coefficient "Beta") and the aforementioned six factors are summarized in Figure 7.11. The abbreviations for the factors are as follows: "UrbRatio" for urbanization ratio with values in the range 0–1; "Popden" for density of population over 65 in persons per km^2; "Income" for median household income in \$10,000; "Poverty" for poverty rate for population over 65 with values in the range 0–1; and "HHI" and "LI", abbreviations stated above, with values 0–1. The mean travel times in the 43 CSAs are negatively correlated with the friction coefficients with a correlation coefficient of -0.62. That is to say, the two measures are generally consistent, but also offer distinctive decay effects. As discussed in Chapter 3, the mean travel time is simply the average time without any indication of the distribution of samples, and the distance decay coefficient is an analytical parameter capturing the declining gradient in the distribution of service volumes in response to increasing distances. The former is straightforward, but cannot capture the specific distribution, and the latter reveals an underlying distribution pattern, but its reliability depends on the function's fitting power. Both help us understand the variability of patient spatial behaviors.

As shown in Figure 7.11, the negative correlations between mean travel time and three of the factors (urbanization ratio, density, and income) are statistically significant. Correspondingly, the positive correlations between distance friction coefficient and two of the factors (urbanization ratio and income) remain statistically significant, but not with the factor "density". Note that the friction coefficient is also negatively related to LI. In other words, a higher localization ratio (more patients seeking services within a delineated CSA)

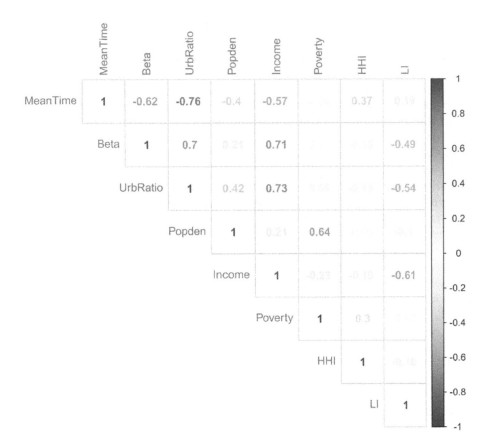

	MeanTime	Beta	UrbRatio	Popden	Income	Poverty	HHI	LI
MeanTime	1	-0.62	-0.76	-0.4	-0.57		0.37	0.19
Beta		1	0.7	0.21	0.71			-0.49
UrbRatio			1	0.42	0.73			-0.54
Popden				1	0.21	0.64		
Income					1	-0.23		-0.61
Poverty						1	0.3	
HHI							1	
LI								1

FIGURE 7.11
Correlation coefficient matrix of variables in the 43 CSAs. (The fading values represent being statistically insignificant at the 0.01 level.)

is associated with a smaller friction coefficient. The mean travel time or the friction coefficient is weakly associated with poverty rate.

Finally, an exploratory multivariate regression is conducted to examine the collective effects of the factors on the distance decay measures. To eliminate insignificant variables and overcome collinearity problems (as revealed in Figure 7.11), a stepwise regression is employed, which yields the result as follows:

$$\text{MeanTime} = 61.34 - 0.02\,\text{Popden} - 3.14\,\text{Income} + 22.41\,\text{HHI, with } R^2 = 0.49$$

$$\text{Beta} = 0.01 + 0.005\,\text{Income, with } R^2 = 0.50$$

where all remaining explanatory variables are statistically significant at the 0.05 level and have variation inflation factors smaller than 1 and thus no collinearity problems among explanatory variables in the model.

The regressions for mean travel time and friction coefficient have similar explanatory power at about 50%. In the model for the mean travel time, three factors such as density of population over 65, median household income, and HHI are statistically significant, and their combination explains 49% of its variation across the 43 CSAs. LI is not significant in correlation with mean travel time (as shown in Figure 7.11), and it is also eliminated from the stepwise regression. In the model for the distance friction parameter, only median household income is retained, and this lone factor has a slightly higher explanatory power (50%). Other factors such as urbanization ratio and LI, though significant in correlation with the friction coefficient, are eliminated due to their collinearity with median household income (as shown in Figure 7.11). In both models, income stands out as the most significant factor as a higher income in a CSA tends to lower its mean travel time and increase its distance friction parameter. This is consistent with the literature (Fotheringham, 1981) that better-developed areas enjoy better infrastructures in health care and transportation, both of which help reduce travel burden reflected in shorter travel time and higher friction coefficient. A CSA with a higher population density tends to have high concentrations in both residents and health care facilities, which reduce its mean travel time, and a higher HHI is associated with a more concentrated health care market (or dominated by a small number of major providers) and thus helps drive up the mean travel time. However, neither density nor HHI exerts such an effect on the friction coefficient. The discrepancy in the effects of these two factors on mean travel time and friction coefficient merits more in-depth future research.

7.5 Summary

This chapter applied some of the techniques introduced in other chapters, such as the distance decay effect and the network community detection methods, in delineating the service areas of a specialized health care, cancer care. It also discussed a method of interpolating suppressed OD flow data by a gravity model, a common challenge for similar tasks involving medical data of small numbers. All are illustrated in a case study in the nine-state Northeast Region of the USA.

All cancer services including cancer-directed surgical procedures, chemotherapy, and radiation treatment are extracted for Medicare patients. Data are then aggregated to the ZIP code area level, and a network composed of ZIP code centroids as nodes and service volumes as edge weights is formed. A three-step process is designed to interpolate suppressed service volumes with values less than 11: (1) A gravity-based regression model is derived by fitting the observed service volumes between ZIP code areas, where the best-fitting distance decay function is identified, (2) the empirically derived model is used to estimate preliminary values for suppressed service volumes, and (3) the preliminarily estimated values are further adjusted by a monotonic transformation to fit within the feasible range [1, 10].

The spatially constrained Louvain and Leiden methods, termed ScLouvain and ScLeiden, are implemented to delineate the CSAs. By "spatially constrained", both algorithms enforce (1) spatial adjacency for each derived CSA, (2) connecting geographic islands to mainland, (3) merging an orphan area to its neighboring CSA, and (4) ensuring the minimum population size for all CSAs. The derived CSAs enjoy higher LI, more compact shape, and more balanced region size than their HRR counterparts. Between the two methods, the ScLeiden method outperforms the ScLouvain method in generating CSAs that are more coherent (with higher LI) and more balanced in size.

The distance decay effect is analyzed by the complementary cumulative distribution functions across CSAs. For most of the CSAs, the exponential function is the best-fitting one. Several factors help explain the variability of distance decay effect, measured in mean travel time and distance friction coefficient, across the CSAs. In short, the mean travel time is negatively related to population density and income and positively associated with the market concentration index (HHI). In other words, cancer patients in CSAs that are more densely settled, are wealthier, and have a less concentrated (thus more competitive) health care market tend to experience shorter travel time on average. The distance decay (travel friction) coefficient tends to be higher in wealthier CSAs.

Appendix A: User Guide: Estimating a Large OD Drive Time Matrix

A.1 Background and Purposes

This user guide is to support the release of data and toolkits related to the following paper: Hu, Y., C. Wang, R. Li, and F. Wang. 2020. Estimating a large drive time matrix between zip codes in the United States: A differential sampling approach. *Journal of Transport Geography* 86, 102770. Users can download the data and toolkit from this website: https://geonavilab. geog.ufl.edu/ downloads/.

The paper illustrated the challenges of estimating a large drive time matrix faced by researchers from various fields, such as geography, public health, and transportation, and proposed a feasible and efficient solution to the estimation of a large drive time matrix from 32,840 origin (O) ZIP codes to 32,840 destination (D) ZIP codes in the USA. The task is broken down to estimation of travel time matrices at three levels. Each begins with a preliminary baseline estimation:

1. Level 1 utilizes a complete road network including interstates, highways, major roads, and local roads to calculate a drive time and/or distance matrix for short-range trips.
2. Level 2 utilizes a simplified road network of only interstates and highways to measure the drive time/or distance matrix for medium-range trips.
3. Level 3 utilizes the geodesic distance to measure the long-range trips.

A subset of OD pairs from each level is then randomly selected, and the drive times for these OD pairs are estimated via the Google Maps API. Based on the regression models between the baseline estimates and the Google times from this subset, we derive the final estimates for the full dataset of ZIP-to-ZIP drive time matrix.

This user guide helps users to implement four tasks:

1. Download our calibrated datasets at Level 1 (0–3 hour drive time) and Level 2 (3–6 hour drive time).
2. Replicate the drive time estimation between ZIP codes in different years and/or different regions.

3. Replicate the drive time estimation between other geographic units, such as census tract and county.

4. Extract a subset of OD ZIP code pairs from our calibrated dataset.

A.2 Data and Programs

The folder "Large _ OD _ Data _ Estimation" contains data and program tools such as:

1. ZCTA _ PWC.gdb: It contains one feature class ZCTA _ PWC _ 2010. It includes 32,840 ZIP code population-weighted centroids calibrated from the population data at the census block level. It has four important fields, ZCTA5CE10, POINT _ X, POINT _ Y, and ST _ NAME, to represent the unique ID of ZIP code, longitude, latitude, and state.

2. NA _ OD _ 0-3hours.csv: It represents the calibrated OD drive time matrix at Level 1 in (0,3] hours.

3. NA _ OD _ 3-6hours.csv: It represents the calibrated OD matrix at Level 2 in (3,6] hours.[1]

4. Generate OD Cost Pro.tbx: It is implemented in ArcGIS Pro to estimate OD drive time and extract calibrated data. Detailed descriptions are provided in the next section.

5. LargeODcost: It contains the Python scripts used in Generate OD Cost Pro.tbx.

6. US _ OD _ Cost _ Calibrated _ Data: It contains two folders, hour03 and hour36, to store the OD matrices at Levels 1 and 2 in ".data" format for fast retrieval.[2] They will be used in the tool Generate OD Cost Pro.tbx to extract a subset of the OD matrices.

The NA _ OD _ 0-3hours.csv and NA _ OD _ 3-6hours.csv have identical fields such as:

- OZCTA: origin ZIP code, identical to the field ZCTA5CE10 in ZCTA _ PWC _ 2010.

- DZCTA: destination ZIP code, identical to the field ZCTA5CE10 in ZCTA _ PWC _ 2010.

---

[1] In rare (188) cases, applying the regression models yielded negative values for estimated distances. We used the original values plus the intrazonal distances to adjust the estimated distances.

[2] Under the two folders, each subfolder is named by the first three digits of the origin ZIP code. Under each subfolder, each file name ended with .data is named by the last two digits of the origin ZIP code, and each record contains the five-digit destination ZIP code, travel time in minutes, and travel distance in miles.

- EstTime: travel time from origin ZIP code to destination ZIP code, unit: minutes.
- EstDist: travel distance from origin ZIP code to destination ZIP code, unit: miles.

The OD drive time matrix data at Level 3 is not provided here due to its massive data size and long processing time for downloading. It can be reconstructed by using the regression model reported in the paper and based on geodesic distances that can be quickly derived by the tool "Generate Near Table" in ArcGIS Pro or the ninth tool (05B Write All OD Pairs with Geodesic Distance) to be discussed in the next section.

A.3 Descriptions of Tools under "Generate OD Cost Pro.tbx"

The section illustrates how to use each tool in "Generate OD Cost Pro.tbx" to estimate, calibrate, and extract an OD drive time matrix by ArcGIS Pro from a road network and by Google Maps API.

In ArcGIS Pro, under Catalog view, right-click Toolboxes and click Add Toolbox to open the dialog window, select and add the toolkit of "Generate OD Cost Pro.tbx" from the folder Large _ OD _ Data _ Estimation. Expand the toolkit to display 12 tools:

1. 00 Set Default Network Setting
2. 01 Snap Point to Road Network (Optional)
3. 02 Slice Feature Layer
4. 03A Generate OD Matrix from Road Network
5. 03B Generate OD Matrix from Google Maps (Optional)
6. 04A Calibrate Inter-zonal OD Matrix (Optional)
7. 04B Calibrate Intra-zonal OD Matrix (Optional)
8. 05A Merge OD Matrix at the Same Level (Optional)
9. 05B Write All OD Pairs with Geodesic Distance
10. 06A Construct OD Pair by States
11. 06B Construct OD Pair by ZCTA list
12. 07 Extract Calibrated Travel Cost using OD pairs

Tools (1)–(9) are used to generate a large OD travel cost matrix (including travel time, distance, or both). Tools (10)–(12) are mainly used to extract the travel cost matrix of the input OD pairs from the calibrated ZIP-to-ZIP pairs illustrated in our paper.

Two important tasks should be done before using these tools. One is to ensure the Script File of each tool points to the same Python script under the folder LargeODcost. To do this, right-click each tool and select Properties to open the dialog window of Tool Properties. In General tab, verify the path of Script File. Another is to create and build a network dataset to ensure it has two costs to represent the travel time and distance. Detailed descriptions are provided in Sub-section 2.2.2 of Chapter 2 or by clicking this link: https://pro.arcgis.com/en/pro-app/latest/help/analysis/networks/how-to-create-a-usable-network-dataset.htm.

Metadata for each tool is included so that users can browse the description of each item in each tool to learn more details. The following provides a brief description of each tool.

1. 00 Set Default Network Setting

   This tool is to set default network environment (Figure A.1). It is necessary when estimating distance and/or travel time at Level 1 and Level 2 with a complete road network for short-range trips and only major highways for medium-range trips, respectively. In other words, it should be run twice with two different network datasets if both levels are used for estimation. For Level 3 to calculate the geodesic distance for the long-range trips, no need to use this tool.

2. 01 Snap Point To Road Network (Optional)

   The optional tool is used for snapping ZIP code point features to the nearest edge of the provided polyline road network within a

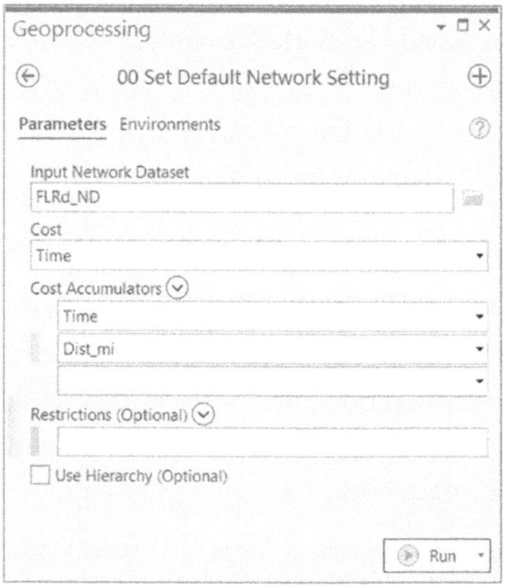

FIGURE A.1
Interface for default network environment setting.

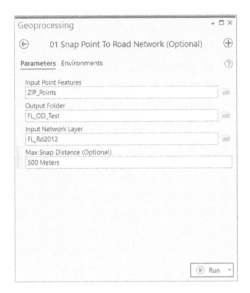

FIGURE A.2
Interface for "Snap Point to Road Network (Optional)" setting.

specific distance. It automatically projects two features into the identical coordinate system. As shown in Figure A.2, the Output Folder should be created by users and the optional Max Snap Distance has a default value of 500 meters. This tool will create a temporary geodatabase named temp.gdb under the output folder.

3. 02 Slice Feature Layer

This tool is to slice the total number of the input point features into multiple features with the same field attributes. The purpose is to speed up the data processing, particularly when the data are large. In other words, if the point feature layer is small, no need to use this tool. Figure A.3 shows the interface. Note that the output GDB should be an empty geodatabase and each generated feature class ends with, for example, _0, _200, and _400 if the number of features in each is 200 for an input feature of 600 points.

4. 03A Generate OD Matrix from Road Network

This tool is to generate an OD cost matrix between points based on the default network setting in the first tool (Figure A.4). If the first tool has not been used, do not leave the last four items blank in this tool. If the input road network dataset is a complete road network with all levels of roads, input 150 for Max Search Distance (equivalent to 180 minutes at the speed of 50 mph); this tool will then generate OD cost matrix at Level 1 (0–3hours). If the input road network dataset is a simplified road network with major highways, input 300 for Max Search Distance (=6 hours), this tool will generate OD cost

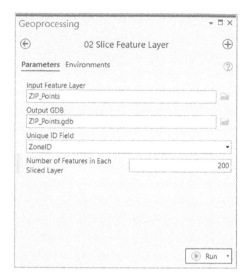

FIGURE A.3
Interface for "Slice Feature Layer" setting.

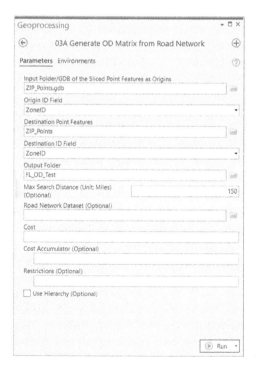

FIGURE A.4
Interface for "Generate OD Matrix from Road Network".

matrix at Level 2 (0–6hours). If users want to calculate the geodesic distances between OD pairs at Level 3, no need to use this tool. Note that Level 1 and Level 2 may have some overlapping records in terms of the composite form of the origin and destination ID fields with non-zero travel times and distances. When using the "05B Write All OD Pairs with Geodesic Distance", only the records at Level 1 will be retained. If the OD cost matrix is computed between the input point features, the Destination Point Features should be a full layer of the input point features without slicing. For example, ZIP _ Points.gdb for Input Folder/GDB contains all sliced feature classes and ZIP _ Points for Destination Point Features refers to the same one without slicing.

5. 03B Generate OD Matrix from Google Maps (Optional)

This tool is to generate OD cost matrix based on the Google Maps Distance Matrix API that provides travel time and distance for a set of origins and a set of destinations (Figure A.5). There might be two scenarios to use this tool. One is to obtain OD cost matrix from Google Maps based on the addresses of origins and destinations and to use the derived travel costs directly. Another is to use an existing OD cost matrix from Google Maps to adjust the one preliminarily derived from a road network. Users need to run related bivariate regression models and sampling and input the two coefficients from

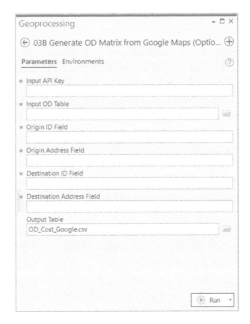

FIGURE A.5
Interface for "Generate OD Matrix from Google Maps (Optional)".

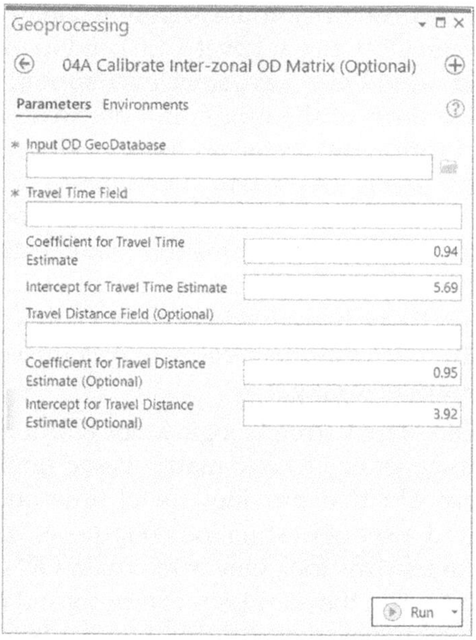

FIGURE A.6
Interface for "Calibrate Inter-zonal OD Matrix (Optional)".

the regression models in the calibration tool. If users prefer to use the default coefficients calibrated from Hu et al. (2020), no need to use this tool.

6. 04A Calibrate Inter-zonal OD Matrix (Optional)

The optional tool is to calibrate the preliminary inter-zonal OD cost matrix at Level 1 and Level 2 by the travel cost matrix from Google Maps, respectively. As shown in Figure A.6, the default values for coefficients and intercepts of travel time and distance are from Hu et al. (2020). Users can also define these parameters based on their own regression models. One scenario for the usage is to calibrate the travel time and/or distance at Level 1 from the tool of "03A Generate OD Matrix from Road Network" by default values. Users are required to set the coefficients and intercepts if the OD cost matrix at Level 2 is calibrated.

7. 04B Calibrate Intra-zonal OD Matrix (Optional)

The optional tool is to calibrate the intra-zonal OD matrix by the perimeter and area size of the input polygon features. As shown in Figure A.7, the default values for the coefficients and intercepts of travel time and distance are derived from Hu et al. (2020). Users can append this intra-zonal OD matrix to the inter-zonal OD matrix derived from the tool of "05B Write All OD Pairs with Geodesic Distance" to obtain a more accurate estimate of the

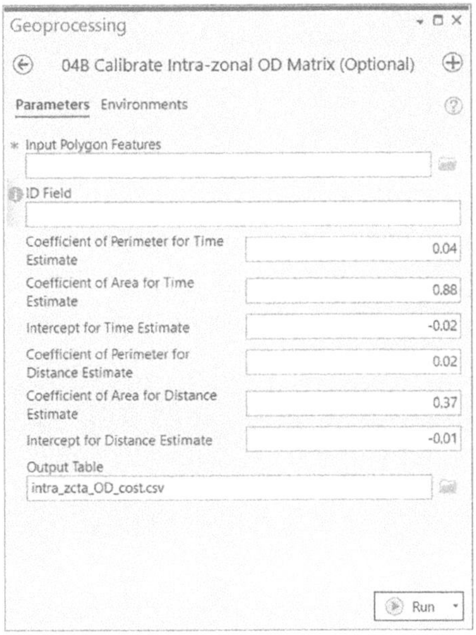

FIGURE A.7
Interface for "Calibrate Intra-zonal OD Matrix (Optional)".

OD drive time matrix, especially for those short-range OD pairs (Hu et al., 2020, p.5).

8. 05A Merge OD Matrix at the Same Level (Optional)

The optional tool is to merge all previously sliced OD cost matrices to one matrix at the same level (Figure A.8). For example, there are three sliced OD matrices estimated at Level 1, use this tool to merge them to one matrix at Level 1; if the sliced OD matrices are at Level 2, use this tool to merge them to one at Level 2.

9. 05B Write All OD Pairs with Geodesic Distance

This tool is to merge the inter-zonal OD cost matrix at Level 1 and Level 2 and calculate the geodesic distances for remaining OD pairs at Level 3. As designed in Hu et al. (2020), if the travel time and/or distance for an OD pair is not found at Level 1, it goes to Level 2, and then to Level 3 to extract the travel cost. As shown in Figure A.9, the default value Name for the first item is generated by the tool of "03A Generate OD Matrix from Road Network" and corresponds to the composite form of Origin ID Field and Destination ID Field with a connection symbol " - ". Users need to input two geodatabases of OD matrices at Level 1 and Level 2, respectively. Note that each feature class in the two geodatabases must have the identical fields representing the origin ID field and destination ID field, respectively. The remaining OD pairs not

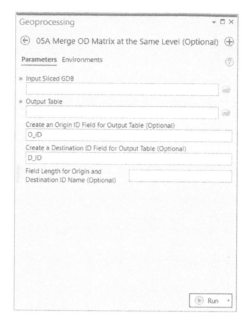

FIGURE A.8
Interface for "Merge OD Matrix at the Same Level (Optional)".

found at Level 1 and Level 2 will be computed based on the latitude (Y Field) and longitude (X Field) of the input ZCTA point or polygon features, i.e., the feature class ZCTA _ PWC _ 2010 under ZCTA _ PWC.gdb. The ZIP code field should be identical to the origin ID field and destination ID field in the two geodatabases. If users only want to obtain OD cost matrix at Levels 1, 2, and 3 without any calibration, select the original estimated travel time and distance for Level 1 and Level 2 and select the default value No for the Calibrate OD Travel Cost (see Figure A.9a). If users want to obtain a calibrated OD cost matrix at three levels, select the calibrated travel time and distance for Level 1 and Level 2 and select Yes for the Calibrate OD Travel Cost. Then the default values for the coefficients and intercepts in Hu et al. (2020) will be shown in this tool (see Figure A.9b).

A.4 Extracting ZIP-to-ZIP OD Cost Matrix

10. 06A Construct OD Pair by States
    This tool is to generate OD pairs with origin ZIP codes and the associated geographic coordinates, destination ZIP codes and the

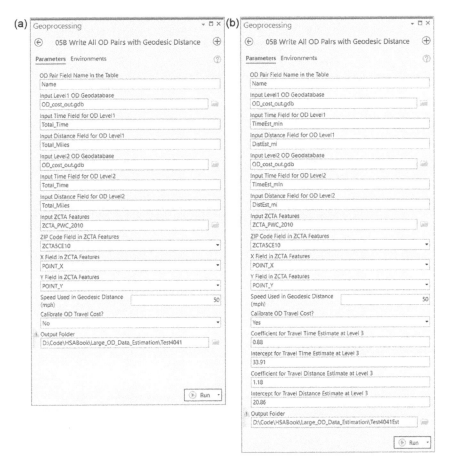

FIGURE A.9
Interfaces for writing (a) all uncalibrated OD pairs and (b) all calibrated OD pairs.

associated geographic coordinates in selected states. The derived OD pairs will be input in the tool of "07 Extract Calibrated Travel Cost using OD pairs" to obtain the calibrated travel time and distance (see Figure A.12). As shown in Figure A.10, the ZCTA_PWC_2010 (N=32,840) contains four fields ZCTA5CE10, ST_NAME, POINT_X, and POINT_Y, and say, users want to create OD pairs between ZIP codes in Florida and Louisiana. The output table will have all OD ZIP code pairs in these two states.

11. 06B Construct OD Pair by ZCTA list
    This tool is to generate OD pairs with origin ZIP codes and the associated geographic coordinates, destination ZIP codes and the associated geographic coordinates based on a list of ZIP codes. As shown in Figure A.11, the input ZCTA list should have a ZIP code

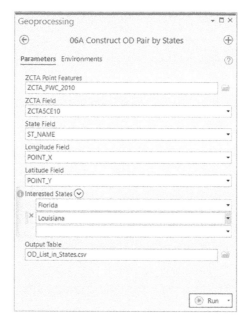

FIGURE A.10
Interface for "Construct OD Pair by States".

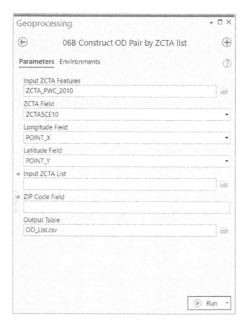

FIGURE A.11
Interface for "Construct OD Pair by ZCTA list".

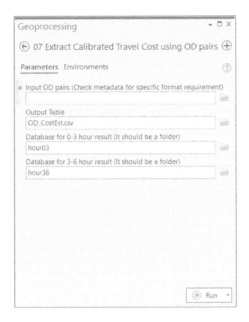

FIGURE A.12
Interface for "Extract Calibrated Travel Cost using OD pairs".

field that corresponds to the ZCTA field in the input ZCTA features. Only the matched OD pairs will be generated, and users can then use the tool "07 Extract Calibrated Travel Cost using OD pairs" to obtain the calibrated travel time and distance (see Figure A.12). For those unmatched ZIP codes, refer to Hu et al. (2020, p. 8).

12. 07 Extract Calibrated Travel Cost using OD pairs

This tool is to extract the calibrated OD travel time and distance from our provided dataset. For those not found at Level 1 or Level 2, this tool will regard them to be OD pairs at Level 3 and automatically compute the geodesic distance and travel time at the speed of 50 mph, and then calibrate them by both the regression models reported in Hu et al. (2020, p. 8). As shown in Figure A.12, the databases for 0–3 hours and 3–6 hours correspond to the subfolder hour03 and hour36 under the folder US _ OD _ Cost _ Calibrated _ Data. The input OD pairs can be those generated from the tools of "06A Construct OD Pair by States" or "06B Construct OD Pair by ZCTA list" or pre-existing OD data that contain fields OZCTA, DZCTA, olat, olong, dlat, and dlong accordingly. For those unmatched OD pairs, refer to Hu et al. (2020, p. 8). Note that it may be time-consuming for a large OD pair dataset. For example, for Florida and Louisiana, our experiment took 1 hour and 7 minutes.

Appendix B: User Guide: How to Create Curved-Line and Straight-Line Network Flow Maps

This user guide introduces how to use ArcGIS Pro to create a straight-line network flow map shown in Figure 4.9a–c in Chapter 4 and how to use Gephi to create a curved-line network flow map shown in Figure 6.8a and b in Chapter 6.

B.1 Data and Tools

The subfolder "ODFlowData" under the folder Florida contains the following data:

1. ZIP_Points.csv: A node file for the network of hospitalization flows with 983 records to represent 983 ZIP code points. The node file contains fields ID, XCoord, YCoord, ZipCode, and POPU that are identical to the fields ZoneID, XCoord, YCoord, ZipCode, and POPU in feature class ZIP_Points under FL_HSA.gdb. Note that the first three fields are required to represent the unique ID and geographic coordinates of each node. The node file is used to create a curved-line network flow map.

2. OD_All_Flows37180.csv: An edge file for the network of hospitalization flows with 37,180 records including edges from a node to itself. The edge file contains fields Source, Target, Weight, Patient_ZipCode, and Hosp_ZipCode that are identical to the fields PatientZipZoneID, Hosp_ZoneID, AllFlows, Patient_ZipCode, and Hosp_ZipCode in table OD_All_Flows under FL_HSA.gdb. The Source and Target fields are also identical to the ID field in the node file. Note that the first three fields are required to represent the origin ID field, destination ID field, and edges between any two nodes. The edge file is used to create a curved-line network flow map.

3. OD_All_Flows: A table under FL_HSA.gdb that contains fields: (1) geographic coordinates XCoord and YCoord for an origin node (ZIP code) represented by field PatientZipZoneID, (2) geographic coordinates Hosp_X_MC and Hosp_Y_MC for a destination

node (hospital) represented by field `Hosp _ ZoneID`, and (3) field `AllFlows` to represent the edges between them. This table is used to create a straight-line network flow map.

4. `ZIP _ Points`: A point feature under `FL _ HSA.gdb` that represents population-weighted centroids of ZIP code areas in Florida. It is used to locate a curved-line network flow map in ArcGIS Pro.

5. `Sd _ 18HSAs _ ROP88`: A feature class under `FL _ HSA _ Results. gdb` in `Results` folder to represent 18 HSAs derived from the ScLeiden method with the global optimal modularity. It has fields `HSAID`, `LI`, `POPU`, and `EstTime`. It is used to be overlaid with curved-line network flows in a map in ArcGIS Pro.

Gephi is an open-source software for network analysis and visualization. It can be downloaded from https://gephi.org/users/download/ and installed in Windows, Mac OS X, or Linux. We also provide the installable files under the subfolder "ODFlowData". Gephi can create a network flow map of either curved or straight lines with different colors and thicknesses, and here it is used to create curved ones. The tool of "XY To Line" in ArcGIS Pro is used to create a network flow map of straight lines.

B.2 Creating a Curved-Line Network Flow Map in Gephi

One important plugin for creating a curved-line network flow map is Geo Layout in Gephi. It can display the graph (network) based on geographic coordinates (i.e., latitude and longitude) and standard projections (i.e., Mercator and Transverse Mercator). The geographic coordinates must be in a numeric data type.

B.2.1 Installing Geo Layout

Open Gephi, and click Tools Menu to open the Plugins dialog window. Click Available Plugins tab, check Geo Layout plugin, and click Install. Follow the instructions to install Geo Layout. Ignore warnings and continue. In the Plugin Installer dialog window, check Restart Now and click Finish to restart Gephi.

B.2.2 Importing the Nodes Data

Click File Menu, select Import Spreadsheet, choose `ZIP _ Points.csv`, and click open to activate the dialog window of "Spreadsheet (CSV)".

Ensure that the Separator is Comma, the import csv file is Nodes table, and Charset is UTF-8, and click Next. Check each field and select its appropriate data type, and click Finish to enter another dialog window of Import report. The node file has 983 nodes. Select Directed for Graph Type[1], and check New workspace. Click OK to close the dialog window, and enter the interface of Data Table tab under Workspace. If no Data Table is shown, click Window Menu and select Data Table. Figure B.1 shows all 983 nodes in Nodes tab.

B.2.3 Importing the Edges Data

Click Edges tab at the right side of Nodes, click Import Spreadsheet, select `OD_All_Flows37180.csv` and click Open to enter the dialog window of "Spreadsheet (CSV)". Similarly, ensure that the Separator is Comma, the import csv file is Edges table, and Charset is UTF-8, and click Next. Check all fields and select the appropriate data type for each field; click Finish to enter another dialog window of Import report. It shows there are 983 nodes and 37,180 edges. Select Directed for Graph Type and Append to existing workspace. Click OK to close the dialog window, and enter the interface of Data Table tab under Workspace. Figure B.2 shows all records in Edges tab.

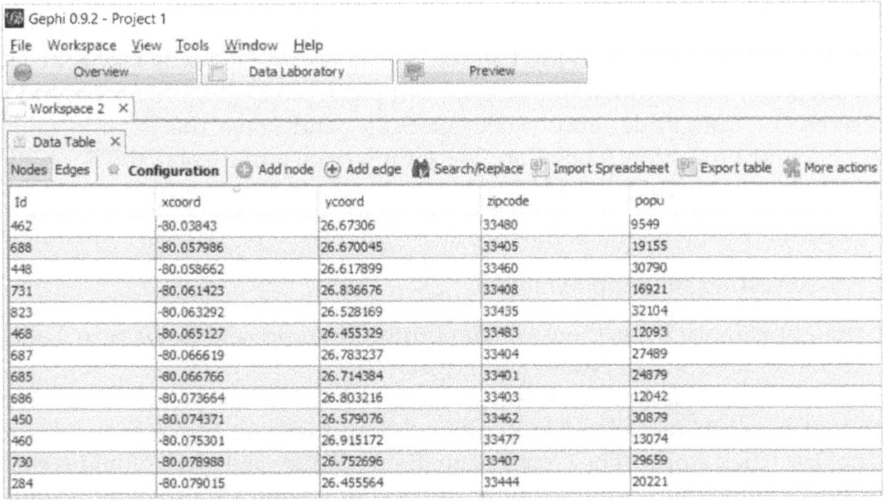
Gephi 0.9.2 - Project 1
File Workspace View Tools Window Help
Overview
Data Laboratory
Preview
Workspace 2
Data Table
Nodes Edges Configuration Add node Add edge Search/Replace Import Spreadsheet Export table More actions
Id xcoord ycoord zipcode popu
462 -80.03843 26.67306 33480 9549
688 -80.057986 26.670045 33405 19155
448 -80.058662 26.617899 33460 30790
731 -80.061423 26.836676 33408 16921
823 -80.063292 26.528169 33435 32104
468 -80.065127 26.455329 33483 12093
687 -80.066619 26.783237 33404 27489
685 -80.066766 26.714384 33401 24879
686 -80.073664 26.803216 33403 12042
450 -80.074371 26.579076 33462 30879
460 -80.075301 26.915172 33477 13074
730 -80.078988 26.752696 33407 29659
284 -80.079015 26.455564 33444 20221

FIGURE B.1
983 ZIP codes in Nodes tab in Gephi.

[1] Users can also select Undirected or Mixed to create other types of graph.

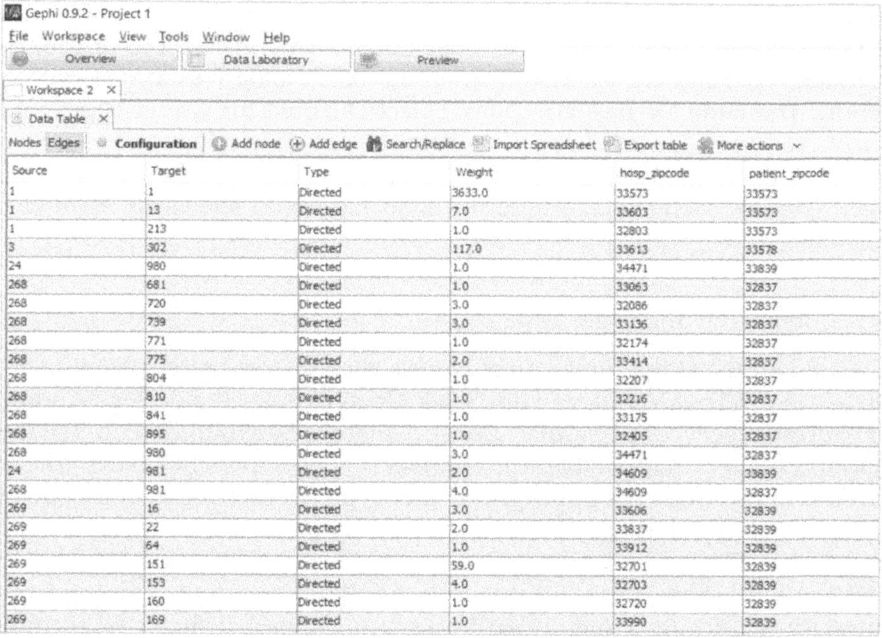

FIGURE B.2
37,180 edges between 983 nodes in Edges tab in Gephi.

B.2.4 Generating the Flow Map

Click Overview tab on the top banner. As shown in Figure B.3, select Geo Layout under the Layout module on the left pane, select ycoord for Latitude, xcoord for Longitude, and 15,000 for Scale, and leave the default value Mercator for Projection. Click Run. The Graph pane will display the hospitalization flow network in Florida.

B.2.5 Adjusting the Map Symbols

In the Appearance pane, there are four buttons to represent Color, Size, Label Color, and Label Size of Nodes and Edges.

Click Color for Nodes; the default value is #c0c0c0 in Unique tab. Click Size for Nodes, select "In-degree" in Ranking tab, and set 2 for Min size and 40 for Max size. Click Apply. The Graph pane displays different sizes of nodes that represent incoming flows ending at the nodes. Users can also click Unique tab to set an equal size for each node.

Click Color for Edges, select Weight in Ranking tab, click ⊞ on the right, and select Default to display different color palettes. Here we select the fourth one. Click Apply to display the weight of edges by different colors. To change the edge (line) color, click Spline under Ranking to open the Interpolate

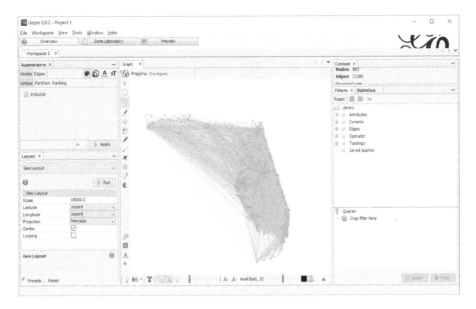

FIGURE B.3
Geo Layout for the network of hospitalization in Gephi.

dialog window. Select the third spline in Templates, and click Close. Click Apply again, and see that the color of edges becomes darker.

Figure B.4 shows all settings for Nodes and Edges in Appearance pane.

Click Preview tab on the top banner, in Preview Settings, check Per_Node Opacity and Show Edges, input 0.5 for Border Width and 0.01 for Thickness of Edges, select Original color, and check Curved for Edges. Click Refresh. The Preview module on the right displays the graph with new settings in Figure B.5. *Users can also uncheck Curved to create straight edges.*

B.2.6 Reducing Insignificant Lines

Click Overview tab on the top banner, expand Edges in the Filters pane on the right, and double-click Edge Weight so that it appears in Queries. The Edge Weight Settings show the edge weight is between 1 and 6,315. Click 1 to select it, change it to 20, and press Enter; then, click Select and Filter button. The insignificant edges of the graph are reduced. Users can also filter edges by different numbers. Click Preview tab on the top banner. Click Refresh to see the graph with significant edges in Figure B.6.

Users can also adjust the settings for the nodes and edges in either Overview or Preview tab. For example, adjust the color of Nodes to be #36A5EB.

B.2.7 Exporting the Map

Click File Menu > Export > SVG/PDF/PNG file… to open the dialog window. Input the File Name, and select PNG Files for Files of type. Click options at

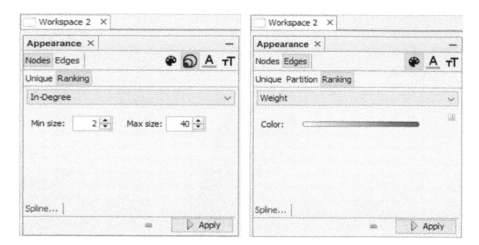

FIGURE B.4
Settings for nodes and edges.

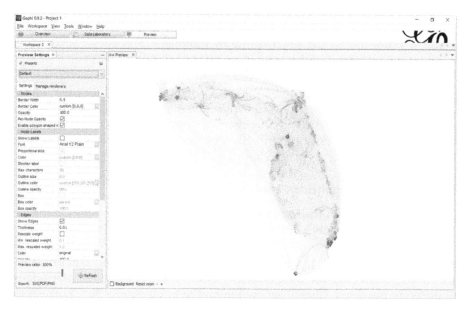

FIGURE B.5
Preview of graph with new settings.

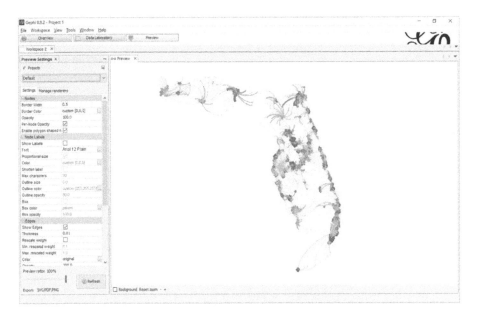

FIGURE B.6
Preview of the graph with significant edges (weight ≥ 20).

the right bottom and set the width, height, margin of the PNG file, and check Transparent background. Click OK. Click Save to export the network flow map. Users can also export the map by clicking "Export: SVG/PDF/PNG" at the bottom of Preview Settings modular under the Preview banner.

B.3 Creating a Straight-Line Network Flow Map in ArcGIS Pro

B.3.1 Creating Lines from OD Coordinates

Open a new project in ArcGIS Pro. In Map view, add the table OD _ All _ Flows under FL _ HSA.gdb and feature class Sd _ 18HSAs _ R0P88 under FL _ HSA _ Results.gdb in the Results folder.

Under Analysis, click Tools to open the Geoprocessing pane. Search the tool "XY To Line", and click it to open the dialog window. As shown in Figure B.7, select OD _ All _ Flows for Input Table, name the output feature class as OD _ All _ Flows _ Line, select XCoord for Start X Field and YCoord for Start Y Field, select Hosp _ X _ MC for End X Field and Hosp _ Y _ MC for End Y Field, leave default values Geodesic for Line Type and GCS_WGS_1984 for Spatial Reference, and check Preserve attributes. Click Run.

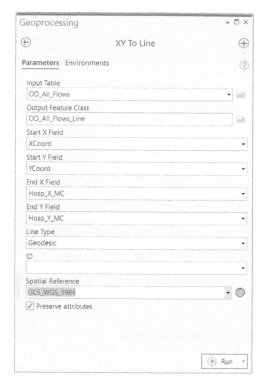

FIGURE B.7
Interface of setting parameters in "XY To Line".

The new feature class OD _ All _ Flows _ Line is automatically loaded in the Contents pane. It has 209,379 (i.e., =983*213) records representing the same number of lines in the map.

B.3.2 Reducing Insignificant Lines

Right-click the feature OD _ All _ Flows _ Line, and select Properties to open the dialog window. In the Layer Properties window, click Definition Query tab on the left > New definition query, and set AllFlows>=20. Click Apply and then OK to close the dialog window.

Right-click the feature OD _ All _ Flows _ Line again, and select Symbology to open the dialog window. As shown in Figure B.8, select Graduated Symbols for Primary symbology and AllFlows for Field, and set the values for Method, Classes, Minimum size, and Maximum size. Users can also click the Template to choose a line symbol.

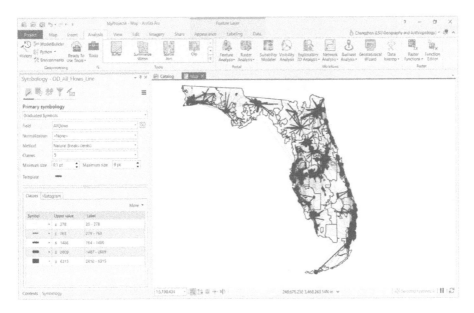

FIGURE B.8
Symbology for straight-line network flow map overlaid with 18 ScLeiden-derived HSAs.

B.3.3 Finalizing the Map

Right-click the feature class Sd _ 18HSAs _ R0P88, and select Symbology. Select Graduated Colors for Primary symbology, LI for Field, 4 for Classes, and White to Black for Color scheme. Input appropriate values in Upper value, and set Label for each range, as shown in Figure 6.8b. Users can also add the layer Hosp _ ZIP, and set parameters for Symbology.

Click either the network flow map or Sd _ 18HSAs _ R0P88, and select Appearance tab. Users can set parameters in Transparency and Layer Blend for two layers. For the network flow map, users can also set the Stretch Type, Resampling Type, and DRA in the Rendering group.

Click Insert tab > New Layout, and click Map Frame to add all three layers. Add legend, north arrow, and scale bar to the layout. Click Share tab > Layout to export the map.

B.4 Creating a Curved-Line Network Flow Map in ArcGIS Pro

This section illustrates how to utilize the curved-line network flows generated in Gephi and overlay it with delineated HSAs in ArcGIS Pro.

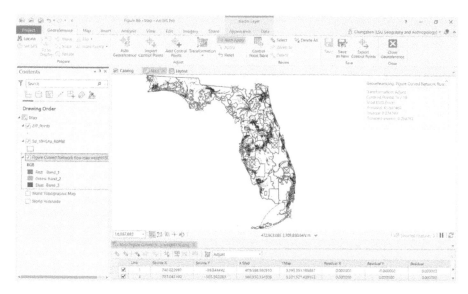

FIGURE B.9
Georeference interface for defining control points in ArcGIS Pro.

Open a new project in ArcGIS Pro. In Contents pane, add two feature classes ZIP _ Points and Sd _ 18HSAs _ ROP88. Load the network flow map as a raster layer. To make the raster layer placed with the current map display of two layers, click the network flow map to select it. In the Imagery tab, click Georeference to open the Georeference tab. Click Fit to Display. The Move, Scale, and Rotate can also be used to adjust the raster layer.

To ensure that the two layers match well, in the Adjust group, click Add Control Points. Select a black dot in the raster layer as a "From point (source)" and click it; find the corresponding point in the ZIP _ Points layer and click it as a "To point (target)". Repeat this step until at least 3 control points are made and evenly distributed across the study area. Users can click Control Point Table in the Review group to verify the residual of each control point and delete unwanted control points with higher residuals and readd control points. Click Transformation and select Adjust, select Auto Apply, and click Save and Close Georeference.

Figure B.9 shows the Georeference interface of control points in two layers. Follow Sub-section B.3.3 to finalize and export the map.

References

Agency for Healthcare Research and Quality (AHRQ). 2011. Healthcare Cost and Utilization Project (HCUP) State Inpatient Databases (SID) - Florida. Rockville, MD. Available www.hcup-us.ahrq.gov/sidoverview.jsp.

Alegana, V. A., C. Khazenzi, S. O. Akech, and R. W. Snow. 2020. Estimating hospital catchments from in-patient admission records: A spatial statistical approach applied to malaria. *Scientific Report* 10, 1324.

Antrim, A. and S. J. Barbeau. 2013. The many uses of GTFS data–opening the door to transit and multimodal applications. Working paper, Center for Urban Transportation Research, University of South Florida.

Bae, S.-H., D. Halperin, J. D. West, M. Rosvall, and B. Howe. 2017. Scalable and efficient flow-based community detection for large-scale graph analysis. *ACM Transactions on Knowledge Discovery from Data* 11, 1–30.

Berry, B. J. L. and R. Lamb. 1974. The delineation of urban spheres of influence: Evaluation of an interaction model. *Regional Studies* 8, 185–190.

Bhatta, B. P. and O. I. Larsen. 2011. Are intrazonal trips ignorable? *Transport Policy* 18, 13–22.

Blondel, V. D., J. L. Guillaume, R. Lambiotte, and E. Lefebvre. 2008. Fast unfolding of communities in large networks. *Journal of Statistical Mechanics: Theory and Experiment* 2008, P10008.

Center for Evaluative Clinical Sciences. 1999. The Dartmouth Atlas of Health Care 1999: The Quality of Medical Care in the United States (edited by J. E. Wennberg). Hanover, NH: Dartmouth Medical School.

Christaller, W. 1966. In C. W. Baskin (trans.), *Central Places in Southern Germany*. Englewood Cliffs, NJ: Prentice-Hall.

Cliff, A. D. and J. K. Ord. 1973. *Spatial Autocorrelation*. London: Pion.

Dartmouth Atlas of Health Care. 2013. *The Dartmouth Atlas of Children's Health Care in Northern New England*. Available https://data.dartmouthatlas.org/downloads/atlases/NNE_Pediatric_Atlas_121113.pdf (last accessed 6-24-2021)

Dartmouth Atlas of Health Care. 2011. *Dartmouth Atlas of Health Care Data HRS-CDR Dataset Documentation*. Available https://hrs.isr.umich.edu/sites/default/files/restricted_data_docs/HRS_CDR_Dartmouth_Atlas_User_Guide.pdf (last accessed 6-24-2021)

De Vries J. J., P. Nijkamp, and P. Rietveld. 2009. Exponential or power distance-decay for commuting? An alternative specification. *Environment and Planning A* 41, 461–480.

Delamater P. L., J. P. Messina, S. C. Grady, V. Winkler Prins, and A. M. Shortridge. 2013. Do more hospital beds lead to higher hospitalization rates? A spatial examination of Roemer's Law. *PLoS ONE* 8(2), e54900.

Dijkstra, E. W. 1959. A note on two problems in connection with graphs. *Numerische Mathematik* 1, 269–271.

Escarce, J. J., and K. Kapur. 2009. Do patients bypass rural hospitals? Determinants of inpatient hospital choice in rural California. *Journal of Health Care for the Poor and Underserved* 20, 625–644.

Expert, P., T. S. Evans, V. D. Blondel, and R. Lambiotte. 2011. Uncovering space-independent communities in spatial networks. *Proceedings of the National Academy of Sciences* 108, 7663–7668.

Fisher, E. and J. Skinner. 2013. Making sense of geographic variations in health care: The new IOM report. Health Affairs Blog available at https://www.healthaffairs.org/do/10.1377/hblog20130724.033319/full/.

Fotheringham, A. S. 1981. Spatial structure and distance-decay parameters. *Annals of the Association of American Geographers* 71, 425–436.

Fotheringham, A. S. and D. W. S. Wong. 1991. The Modifiable Areal Unit Problem in multivariate statistical analysis. *Environment and Planning A* 23(7), 1025–1044.

Freeman, L. 1979. Centrality in social networks: Conceptual clarification. *Social Networks* 1, 215–239.

Gao, S., Y. Liu, Y. Wang, and X. Ma. 2013. Discovering spatial interaction communities from mobile phone data. *Transactions in GIS* 17(3), 463–481.

Ghosh, A. and S. McLafferty. 1987. *Location Strategies for Retail and Service Firms.* Lexington, MA: D.C. Heath.

Glover, J. A. 1938. The incidence of tonsillectomy in school children. *Proceedings of the Royal Society of Medicine* 31, 95–113.

Goodman, D. C., S. S. Mick, D. Bott, T. Stukel, C.-H. Chang, N. Marth, J. Poage, and H. J. Carretta. 2003. Primary care service areas: A new tool for the evaluation of primary care services. *Health Services Research* 38, 287–309.

Goodman, D. C., and E. S. Fisher. 2008. Physician workforce crisis? Wrong diagnosis, wrong prescription. *New England Journal of Medicine*, 358(16), 1658–1661.

Goodman D., E. Fisher, C. Chang, N. E. Morden, J. O. Jacobson, K. Murray, and S. Miesfeldt. 2010. *Quality of End-of-Life Cancer Care for Medicare Beneficiaries: Regional and Hospital-Specific Analyses.* Hanover, NH: The Dartmouth Institute for Health Policy & Clinical Practice.

Guo, D. 2008. Regionalization with dynamically constrained agglomerative clustering and partitioning (REDCAP). *International Journal of Geographical Information Science* 22, 801–823.

Halás, M., P. Klapka, and P. Kladivo. 2014. Distance-decay functions for daily travel-to-work flows. *Journal of Transport Geography* 35, 107–119.

Hansen, W. G. 1959. How accessibility shapes land use, *Journal of the American Institute of Planners* 25, 73–76.

Haynes, A. G., M. M. Wertli, and D. Aujesky. 2020. Automated delineation of hospital service areas as a new tool for health care planning. *Health Services Research* 55(3): 469–475.

Hillier, B. 1996. *Space is the Machine: A Configurational Theory of Architecture.* Cambridge: Cambridge University Press.

Horner, M. W. and A. T. Murray. 2002. Excess commuting and the modifiable areal unit problem. *Urban Studies* 39, 131–139.

Hu, Y., C. Wang, R. Li, and F. Wang. 2020. Estimating a large drive time matrix between zip codes in the United States: A differential sampling approach. *Journal of Transport Geography* 86, 102770.

Hu, Y. and F. Wang. 2016. Temporal trends of intraurban commuting in Baton Rouge 1990-2010. *Annals of the American Association of Geographers* 106: 470–479.

Hu, Y. and F. Wang. 2019. *GIS-based Simulation and Analysis of Intra-Urban Commuting.* Boca Raton, FL: CRC Press.

Hu, Y., F. Wang, and I. Xierali. 2018. Automated delineation of hospital service areas and hospital referral regions by modularity optimization. *Health Services Research* 53, 236–255.

Huff, D. L. 1963. A probabilistic analysis of shopping center trade areas. *Land Economics* 39, 81–90.

Huff, D. L. 2003. Parameter estimation in the Huff model. *ArcUser* 2003, 34–36.

Institute of Medicine (IOM). 2013. *Variation in Health Care Spending: Target Decision Making, not Geography.* Washington, D.C.: The National Academies Press.

Institute of Medicine (IOM). 2014. *Innovation in Cancer Care and Implications for Health Systems: Global Oncology Trend Report.* Plymouth Meeting, PA: IMS Institute for Healthcare Informatics.

Jia, P., I. Xierali, and F. Wang. 2015. Evaluating and re-demarcating the Hospital Service Areas in Florida. *Applied Geography* 60, 248–253

Jia, P., F. Wang, and I. Xierali. 2017a. Using a Huff-based model to delineate Hospital Service Areas. *Professional Geographer* 69, 522–530.

Jia, P., F. Wang, and I. Xierali. 2017b. Delineating hierarchical Hospital Service Areas in Florida. *Geographical Review* 107, 608–623.

Jia, P., F. Wang, and I. Xierali. 2019. Differential effects of distance decay on hospital inpatient visits among subpopulations in Florida. *Environmental Monitoring and Assessment* 191(S2), 381.

Jia, P., F. Wang, and I. Xierali. 2020. Evaluating the effectiveness of the Hospital Referral Region (HRR) boundaries: A pilot study in Florida. *Annals of GIS* 26, 251–260.

Kilaru, A. S., D. J. Wiebe, D. N. Karp, J. Love, M. J. Kallan, and B. G. Carr. 2015. Do hospital service areas and hospital referral regions define discrete health care populations? *Medical Care* 53(6), 510–516.

Kuai, X. and F. Wang. 2020. Global and localized neighborhood effects on public transit ridership in Baton Rouge, Louisiana. *Applied Geography* 124, 102338.

Lester, D. 1999. Native American suicide rates, acculturation stress and traditional integration. *Psychological Reports* 84(2), 398–398.

Liberman, N., Y. Trope, and E. Stephan. 2007. Psychological distance. In *Social Psychology: Handbook of Basic Principles* (edited by A. W. Kruglanski and E. T. Higgins, 2nd ed.). New York: Guilford Publications, 353–384.

Liu, Y., F. Wang, C. Kang, Y. Gao, and Y. Lu. 2014. Analyzing relatedness by toponym co-occurrences on web pages. *Transactions in GIS* 18, 89–107.

Luo, W. and F. Wang. 2003. Measures of spatial accessibility to health care in a GIS environment: Synthesis and a case study in Chicago region. *Environment and Planning B-Planning & Design* 30, 865–884.

McLafferty, S. and F. Wang. 2009. Rural reversal? Rural-urban disparities in late-stage cancer risk in Illinois. *Cancer* 115, 2755–2764.

Miami-Dade County Transportation and Public Works. 2019. Ridership Technical Report. Available https://www.miamidade.gov/transit/library/rtr/2019-10-Ridership-Technical-Report.pdf.

Miami-Dade Transportation Planning Organization. 2018. Factors Affecting Transit Ridership in Miami-Dade County Final Report. Available http://www.miami-dadetpo.org/library/studies/factors-affecting-transit-ridership-in-miami-dade-county-final-report-2018-11.pdf.

Mu, L., F. Wang, V. W. Chen, and X. Wu. 2015. A place-oriented, mixed-level regionalization method for constructing geographic areas in health data dissemination and analysis. *Annals of the Association of American Geographers* 105, 48–66.

Nakanishi, M. and L. G. Cooper. 1974. Parameter estimates for multiplicative competitive interaction models—Least square approach. *Journal of Marketing Research* 11, 303–311.

Năstase, I. I., I. Pătru-Stupariu, and F. Kienast. 2019. Landscape preferences and distance decay analysis for mapping the recreational potential of an urban area. *Sustainability* 11, 3620.

National Cancer Institute (NCI). 2014. *ICD-9-CM Casefinding List: International Classification of Diseases.* Available https://seer.cancer.gov/tools/casefinding/case2014.html.

Newman, M. E. J. 2004. Fast algorithm for detecting community structure in networks. *Physical Review E* 69, 066133.

Newman, M. E. J., and M. Girvan. 2004. Finding and evaluating community structure in networks. *Physical Review E* 69, 026113.

Onega, T., J. Alford-Teaster, S. Andrews, C. Ganoe, M. Perez, K. David, and X. Shi. 2014. Why health services research needs geoinformatics: Rationale and case example. *Journal of Health & Medical Informatics,* 5(6), 176.

Onega, T., E. J. Duell, X. Shi, E. Demidenko, and D. Goodman. 2009a. Determinants of NCI Cancer Center attendance in Medicare patients with lung, breast, colorectal, or prostate cancer. *Journal of General Internal Medicine* 24, 205–210.

Onega, T., E. J. Duell, X. Shi, E. Demidenko, D. Gottlieb, and D. C. Goodman. 2009b. Influence of NCI cancer center attendance on mortality in lung, breast, colorectal, and prostate cancer patients. *Medical Care Research and Review* 66, 542–560.

Ozaki, N., H. Tezuka, and M. Inaba. 2016. A simple acceleration method for the Louvain algorithm. *International Journal of Computer and Electrical Engineering* 8, 207–218.

Paskett, E. D. and R. A. Hiatt. 2018. Catchment areas and community outreach and engagement: The new mandate for NCI-designated Cancer Centers. *Cancer Epidemiology, Biomarkers & Prevention* 27(5), 517–519.

Radcliff, T. A., M. Brasure, I. S. Moscovice, and J. T. Stensland. 2003. Understanding rural hospital bypass behavior. *The Journal of Rural Health: Official Journal of the American Rural Health Association and the National Rural Health Care Association* 19, 252–259.

Radley, D. C. and C. Schoen. 2012. Geographic variation in access to care — The relationship with quality. *The New England Journal of Medicine* 367(1), 3–6.

Reichardt, J. and S. Bornholdt. 2006. Statistical mechanics of community detection. *Physical Review E* 74, 1–14.

Reilly, W. J. 1931. *The Law of Retail Gravitation.* New York: Knickerbocker.

Roos, N. P. 1993. Linking patients to hospitals: Defining urban hospital service populations. *Medical Care* 31(5), YS6–YS15.

Rosenberg, B. L., J. A. Kellar, A. Labno, D. H. Matheson, M. Ringel, P. VonAchen, R. I. Lesser, Y. Li, J. B. Dimick, A. A. Gawande, S. H. Larsson, and H. Moses 3rd. 2016. Quantifying geographic variation in health care outcomes in the united states before and after risk-adjustment. *PloS one* 11(12), e0166762.

Sheps Center for Health Services Research. 2021. Rural Hospital Closures: More Information. Available https://www.shepscenter.unc.edu/programs-projects/-rural-health/rural-hospital-closures/ (last accessed 7-26-2021).

Shi, X., J. Alford-Teaster, T. Onega, and D. Wang. 2012. Spatial access and local demand for major cancer care facilities in the United States. *Annals of the Association of American Geographers* 102, 1125–1134.

Taylor, P. J. 1983. Distance decay in spatial interactions. In *Concepts and Techniques in Modern Geography* (edited by the Study Group in Quantitative methods, of the Institute of British Geographers). Norwich, England: Geo Books.

Tobler, W. R. 1970. A computer movie simulating urban growth in the Detroit region. *Economic Geography* 46, 234–240.

Traag, V. A., L. Waltman, and N. J. Van Eck. 2019. From Louvain to Leiden: Guaranteeing well-connected communities. *Scientific Reports* 9, 5233.

Waltman, L., and N. J. Van Eck. 2013. A smart local moving algorithm for large-scale modularity-based community detection. *The European Physical Journal B* 86, 471.

Wang, C., F. Wang, and T. Onega. 2021a. Network optimization approach to delineating health care service areas: Spatially constrained Louvain and Leiden algorithms. *Transactions in GIS* 25, 1065–1081.

Wang C., F. Wang, and T. Onega. 2021b. Spatial behavior of cancer care utilization in distance decay in the Northeast region of the U.S. *Travel Behaviour and Society* 24, 291–302.

Wang, F. 2001. Regional density functions and growth patterns in major plains of China 1982–90. *Papers in Regional Science* 80, 231–240.

Wang, F. 2003. Job proximity and accessibility for workers of various wage groups. *Urban Geography* 24, 253–271.

Wang, F. 2012. Measurement, optimization and impact of health care accessibility: A methodological review. *Annals of the Association of American Geographers* 102, 1104–1112.

Wang, F. 2015. *Quantitative Methods and Socio-Economic Applications in GIS* (2nd edition). Boca Raton, FL: CRC Press.

Wang, F. 2018. Inverted two-step floating catchment area method for measuring facility crowdedness. *Professional Geographer* 70, 251–260.

Wang, F. 2021. From 2SFCA to i2SFCA: integration, derivation and validation. *International Journal of Geographical Information Science* 35, 628–638.

Wang, F., C. Wang, Y. Hu, J. Weiss, J. Alford-Teaster, and T. Onega. 2020. Automated delineation of cancer service areas in northeast region of the United States: A network optimization approach. *Spatial and Spatio-temporal Epidemiology* 33, 100338.

Wang, F. and Y. Xu. 2011. Estimating O-D matrix of travel time by Google Maps API: Implementation, advantages and implications. *Annals of GIS* 17, 199–209.

Ward, M. M., F. Ullrich, K. Matthews, G. Rushton, R. Tracy, D. F. Bajorin, M. A. Goldstein, M. P. Kosty, S. S. Bruinooge, A. Hanley, and C. F. Lynch. 2014. Access to chemotherapy services by availability of local and visiting oncologists. *Journal of Oncology Practice* 10(1), 26–31.

Wennberg, J. and A. Gittelsohn. 1973. Small area variations in health care delivery. *Science* 182 (4117), 1102–1108.

Wilson A. G. 1969. The use of entropy maximizing models in the theory of trip distribution, mode split and route split. *Journal of Transport Economics and Policy* 3, 108–126.

Xu, Y. and F. Wang. 2015. Built environment and obesity by urbanicity in the U.S. *Health & Place* 34, 19–29.

Young, W. J. 2005. Distance decay values and shopping center size. *The Professional Geographer* 27, 304–309.

Zhang, Y., H. Baik Seo, F. A. Mark, and K. Baicker. 2012. Comparing local and regional variation in health care spending. *The New England Journal of Medicine* 367(18), 1724–1731.

Index

absolute error 46
Agency for Healthcare Research and
    Quality (AHRQ) 5
AHA *see* American Hospital Association
    (AHA)
AHRQ *see* Agency for Healthcare
    Research and Quality (AHRQ)
AIC *see* Akaike information criterion
    (AIC)
Akaike information criterion (AIC) 49, 56
alighting time 37
American Hospital Association (AHA)
    5, 63
API key 27–28
ArcGIS Pro 8, 9, 11–15, 19, 21, 27–28, 30, 37,
    70, 73, 77, 92, 94–95, 97–98, 104,
    111–112, 116, 119, 129, 131–132,
    174–175, 187–188, 193, 196
ASCII file 26
aspatial communities 128, 130–131, 159
aspatial leiden method 137, 151
aspatial louvain method 137, 151
aspatial network 128

balanced region size 85, 87–89, 139, 141,
    147–148, 151, 160–161, 171
bed-to-population ratio 107
behavioral distance 13
best-fitting distance decay function
    7, 11, 39, 43–44, 47, 49, 59–60,
    94, 171
bivariate linear regression 45
boarding time 23, 37
breaking point (BP) 101–102
"Build A Spatial Adjacency Matrix" tool
    70, 72, 74, 76–77, 81, 92, 116, 130,
    132, 135
build network tool 16, 23

"calculate regionalization indices" tool
    72, 75, 84
cancer-directed surgical procedure
    154, 170

cancer service areas (CSAs) 2, 122, 125,
    153, 155, 158–164, 166–171
cardiovascular surgery 1, 6, 68–69,
    71–72, 74–75, 77, 79, 81–82, 85,
    88–92, 119, 133–134, 136, 145, 147
cartesian coordinates 11–12
Catalog pane 15, 22, 27
catchment areas (CAs) 1, 2, 4
Centers for Medicare and Medicaid
    Services (CMS) 61, 154–156
centrality indices 13
central place theory 1, 41–42
chemotherapy 154, 170
City of Miami 19
closest facility tool 97
CMS *see* Centers for Medicare and
    Medicaid Services (CMS)
coefficient of determination 46
collinearity 169–170
community detection 7, 9–10, 43, 60, 72,
    119, 121–123, 125, 127, 129–130,
    132–133, 136–137, 139, 142–145,
    149–153, 158–160, 170
complementary cumulative distribution
    curve 39, 49, 53, 55, 166
complementary cumulative distribution
    function 53, 55–56, 60, 171
compound power-exponential function
    41, 59, 115
concatenate field 18–19, 25
connect network dataset transit sources
    to streets tool 22
"consolidate flows at HSA level" tool 70,
    73, 80, 82, 92, 132–133
contents pane 17, 22, 24, 81–82, 95, 97, 129,
    195–196
continuous function 40, 115, 164
correlation coefficient matrix 169
create network dataset from template
    tool 22
create network dataset tool 15
create Thiessen polygons tool 95
CSAs *see* Cancer service areas (CSAs)

csv file format 72–73, 135, 189
curved-line network flow map 141,
        187–188, 196

Dartmouth Atlas of Health Care Project
        1, 9, 61–64, 82, 92
Dartmouth HRRs 1, 3, 68, 73, 84, 88, 90,
        147, 153, 159–160, 162
Dartmouth HSAs 1, 3, 8, 61–64, 73, 75–76,
        82, 84–86, 88, 91, 137, 141–142
Dartmouth Institute for Health Policy &
        Clinical Practice 3
Dartmouth method 8–10, 61, 63–65,
        67–69, 88–93, 111, 116, 119, 122,
        125, 143–144, 150, 152, 160
"Dartmouth Method (HSAs or HRRs)"
        tool 72, 74, 77, 79, 81–82, 92, 116
data suppression 156
decimal degrees 12
demand-based approach (proximal
        areas) 95
dependent variable 46–47, 55
destination ZIP code 33, 36, 64–65, 67, 73,
        78, 81–83, 85–86, 133, 135–136,
        139–140, 142, 168, 174–175,
        182–183
differential sampling method
        (approach) 8, 32, 155, 173
directed network 12
directed weighted network 66
dissolve tool 95, 97–98, 100, 106
distance decay behavior 8, 39, 57, 109,
        153, 163, 165
distance decay effect 9, 39, 41, 43, 45, 47,
        49–50, 52–55, 58, 60, 93, 102–103,
        157, 165–166, 170–171
distance decay function 7–8, 11, 39–45,
        47–49, 52–55, 57, 59–60, 94, 103,
        115, 156–157, 166, 171
distance decay rule 11, 13, 39
distance friction coefficient 41, 45–46, 59,
        102, 108–109, 164, 166–168, 171
drive time matrix 8, 11, 14–15, 21, 32–33,
        37, 173–175, 181

edge effect 4
edge weight 43, 66–67, 123, 125, 127–128,
        155, 157, 170, 191

enclaved node 128
enclosed node 128
estimated flow 43, 74, 116, 118
Euclidean distance 11–12, 14, 37, 93–94,
        96–97, 100–101, 111, 114
Euclidean-distance-based proximal
        area 101
exponential function 41, 49, 59, 115,
        166, 171

fast local move 124–125
first law of geography 8, 11, 39
fixed-route transit service 19
Florida 4, 5, 7–9, 15, 19, 21, 27, 39, 47–51,
        54, 56–58, 60–61, 69–70, 76–77,
        79, 82–83, 86, 88, 90, 92, 94, 96,
        99, 106–108, 110–112, 117, 121,
        129, 131–132, 136, 140, 147, 151,
        183, 185, 187–188, 190
Florida Transit Information System
        (FTIS) 19
functional region 1, 2–3, 93

Garin–Lowry model 46
Gaussian function 41, 49, 115
General Transit Feed Specification
        (GTFS) 19–21, 37
Generate Near Table tool 14, 37, 175
geodatabase 5–6, 19, 21, 28, 46, 69, 73, 77,
        82–84, 133, 135, 177, 181–182
geodesic distance 11–12, 14, 32–34, 36–37,
        94–95, 111–112, 114, 119, 173,
        175–176, 179–181, 185
geographic compactness 74–75, 78, 81,
        83, 85–88, 90, 129, 131, 133, 136,
        139–140, 147, 151, 160
geographic coordinates 12, 20, 73,
        182–183, 187–188
Geographic information systems (GIS) 2,
        4–6, 11–14, 19, 37, 93–94, 97, 104,
        110, 120
geographic island 64–65, 159, 171
geographic island rule 159
geoprocessing pane 15–16, 18, 21–23, 25,
        28, 84, 95, 97, 193
GIS *see* Geographic information systems
        (GIS)
global maximal modularity 130

global optimal modularity 128, 131, 133, 136, 139, 143, 145–146, 149, 188

GNU GPL2 license 70

Google Cloud Platform Console 27

Google Maps API 8, 11, 13, 25, 29–35, 37, 155, 173, 175

Google Maps Distance Matrix API 26, 29, 179

gravitation (gravity model) 101–102

gravity model 9, 43–55, 101, 119, 156, 170

GTFS *see* General Transit Feed Specification (GTFS)

GTFS To Network Dataset Transit Sources tool 21

HCUP *see* Healthcare Cost and Utilization Project (HCUP)

Healthcare Cost and Utilization Project (HCUP) 4–5, 8, 32, 62, 92

Herfindahl–Hirschman Index (HHI) 168–171

HHI *see* Herfindahl–Hirschman Index (HHI)

hierarchal health care system 42

hinterland 2

Hospital service areas (HSAs) 1–5, 7–11, 14, 19, 28, 42–43, 46, 60–94, 97, 101–102, 104, 106–114, 116–119, 121–122, 125, 128–153, 161, 187–188, 193, 195–196

Hospital referral regions (HRRs) 1, 3, 5, 8, 42, 60–63, 67–69, 72–77, 79, 81–85, 88–92, 116, 119, 121, 125, 129–133, 135–137, 139, 145–151, 153, 159–160, 162–164, 171

"HSA Delineation" toolkit 69–70, 77, 84, 116, 129, 131–132

HSAs *see* Hospital service areas (HSAs)

HRRs *see* Hospital referral regions (HRRs)

Huff–Dartmouth Method tool 74, 116, 118

Huff model 7–11, 14, 39, 42, 46–47, 60, 74, 93–94, 101–116, 118–122, 150

igraph package 70

independent variable 47

Institute of Medicine (IOM) 3, 153

Inter-zonal drive time 33–34

Intra-zonal drive time 33, 35–36

inverted two-step floating catchment area (i2SFCA) method 43–44

IOM *see* Institute of Medicine (IOM)

i2SFCA *see* inverted two-step floating catchment area (i2SFCA) method

Join Field tool 18–19, 25

kernel function 40

label setting algorithm 12

large city problem (Dartmouth method) 64–65, 91

large metropolitan 49–50, 52–53, 60

Leiden algorithm 9, 121–122, 124–125, 129, 139, 151, 161, 203

leidenalg package 70

Linear ordinary least square (LOLS) regression 45–47, 49, 60

link impedance 12

LI *see* Localization index (LI)

Localization index (LI) 8, 67–69, 74–75, 78–79, 81–83, 85–90, 92, 116, 118, 129, 131, 133, 136, 139–149, 151, 160–163, 168, 170–171

local nodes moving 123–125, 128

logarithmic transformation 45, 60

log-logistic function 41, 49–50, 52, 56, 60

log-normal function 41, 59

LOLS *see* Linear ordinary least square (LOLS) regression

Louvain algorithm 70, 121–124, 129, 139, 151, 161

Manhattan distance 11–12, 14

maximum hospitalization problem (Dartmouth method) 64–65, 67

mean travel time 166–171

median household income 49–50, 168, 170

Medicaid 1, 5, 56

Medicaid beneficiaries 58–60

medicare 1, 3, 5, 9, 42, 56, 61–63, 68, 91, 168, 170

Medicare beneficiaries 3, 58, 60, 62

Medicare beneficiary denominator file 154

Medicare Parts A and B 154
mental distance 13
Metrobus 19
Metromover 19
metropolitan statistical area 1
Metrorail 19
Miami-Dade County 19–21, 25–28, 30
Miami-Dade County Transportation
    and Public Works 19
Miami-Dade Transportation Planning
    Organization 19
micropolitan 49–50, 52–53, 60
minimum localization index 67, 74, 79,
    81–82, 129
modifiable areal unit problem (MAUP) 2
modularity 43, 122–128, 130–131, 133,
    136–140, 143, 145–149, 151,
    159–160, 188
modularity optimization 123
monotonic transformation 156, 171
Monte Carlo simulation method 35
multiplicative competitive interaction
    (MCI) model 103, 202
multivariate regression 169

National Cancer Institute (NCI) 1, 4, 154
National Cancer Institute (NCI) Cancer
    Center 1
NCI *see* National Cancer Institute (NCI)
near tool 94–95
network aggregation 123–125, 129
network analysis module 15, 19, 37, 94,
    97, 99
network community detection method
    7, 10, 72, 119, 121, 129–130,
    132–133, 136–137, 139, 142–145,
    149, 151–152, 160, 170
"Network Community Detection
    Method (ScLeiden or
    ScLouvain)" tool 72, 129,
    132–133, 136
network dataset 15–16, 19, 21–24, 31,
    176–177
network distance 11–12, 15, 37
network refinement 124–125, 127
network travel time 11–12, 34
NetworkX 70
neurosurgery 1, 6, 68–69, 71–72, 74–75,
    77–82, 85, 88–92, 119, 133–134,
    136, 145, 147–148, 151

New BSD License 69–70
NLLS *see* Nonlinear least square (NLLS)
    regression
non-independent HSA problem
    (Dartmouth method) 64,
    66–67, 91
Nonlinear least square (NLLS)
    regression 46–47, 49, 56, 60
normal function 41, 59
Northeast Region of the USA 9, 122, 125,
    153, 158, 163, 170
npz file format 73, 77, 130
null model 122
NumPy package 73

OD Cost Matrix tool 15–17, 24, 36–37, 98
OD distance matrix 7
OD (origin–destination) flow 5, 9–10, 49,
    93, 94, 104, 114, 119, 170
OD travel time matrix 7, 25, 28–29, 36, 98
onboard travel time 37
online routing app 13
order of service (in the central place
    theory) 42
Origin-Destination Cost Matrix tool 17, 24
orphan node 128, 159
orphan node rule 159
oversampling 34

PAC *see* perimeter-to-area (PAC) ratio
PCSAs *see* Primary care service area
    (PCSAs)
Pediatric surgical areas (PSAs) 1, 62
percentage error 46
perimeter-to-area (PAC) ratio 83, 85–90,
    139–140, 142, 147, 151, 160
planar surface 12
plurality rule 8, 9, 63–64, 68, 89, 91, 93,
    119, 121–122, 150
point ZIP code 63, 154
population-weighted centroids 6, 36, 95,
    97, 154, 174, 188
potential crowdedness 43–44
potential (gravity model) 102,
    104–105, 115
poverty rate 168–169
power function 41, 45, 47–48, 54, 94,
    102–104, 109, 156–157, 166
Primary care service area (PCSAs) 1,
    62, 67

proximal areas 94–101
proximal area method 93–94, 101,
        105, 119
projected coordinate system 26, 28, 74,
        114, 129
projected flow 110
proximal region 2
PSAs *see* Pediatric surgical areas (PSAs)
pseudo-R², 46, 49, 56
psychological distance 13
python package 15, 69, 116, 132
Python package manager
        (ArcGIS Pro) 70
Python program 25

queen contiguity 64–65, 136

R², 30–31, 35, 41, 46–47, 54–55, 156,
        166, 169
R programming 47
radians 12
radiation 154, 170
random neighbor move 124, 126
random network 122
random sampling 32
range (in the central place theory) 42
refined Dartmouth method 7–8, 61,
        63, 66–69, 72, 74, 76–77, 79,
        82, 85–88, 90, 92, 94, 110, 116,
        118–119, 121, 139, 141, 144–146,
        148–149, 151
refined Huff model 9, 103
regionalization 9, 72–73, 75–76, 84–85,
        88, 159
Reilly's law 101–102
resolution parameter (network analysis)
        122–123, 130
Rook contiguity 64

SAS software 47
scalar parameter (in log-logistic
        function) 50
scale-flexible (scale-flexibility) 9, 136,
        144, 151, 159
SciPy 69
ScLeiden *see* Spatially constrained
        Leiden (ScLeiden) method
ScLouvain *see* Spatially constrained
        Louvain (ScLouvain) method
Search Tolerance setting 17, 98

self-loop 67
shape parameter (in log-logistic
        function) 50, 58
Sheps Center for Health Services
        Research 53, 103
shortest-path distance 12
shortest-path travel time 12
shortest-route problem 12
SID *see* State Inpatient Database (SID)
small area analysis 61
small metropolitan 49–50, 52–53, 60
small population sample 156
smart local move 124, 126
social distance 13
spatial accessibility 37, 39, 43, 44, 46
spatial adjacency matrix 64–65, 68,
        70–74, 76–77, 81–82, 92, 116, 128,
        130, 132–133, 135–136, 159
spatial adjacency rule 159
spatial behavior 9, 13, 39, 41–43, 59, 163,
        166, 168
spatial community 128, 159
spatial constraints 9, 43, 125, 129–131,
        137, 151
spatial contiguity 9, 63, 94, 125, 128, 130,
        133, 136–137, 151
spatial impedance 11, 37, 41, 54, 94, 97,
        112, 119
spatial interaction model 39, 43–45, 47,
        49–50, 53, 55, 60
spatial join tool 84, 95, 97
Spatially constrained Leiden (ScLeiden)
        method 9, 72, 121, 125–151, 153,
        158–162, 171, 188, 195
Spatially constrained Louvain
        (ScLouvain) method 9, 72,
        121, 125–126, 128–129, 131–133,
        136–151, 153, 158–162, 171
spatial network 5, 43, 128, 159
Spatial non-contiguity problem
        (Dartmouth method) 64, 66, 92
Specialized hospital 5–6, 60, 68–69, 81,
        88–90, 119
Special Transportation Services (STS) 19
square-root exponential function 41, 45,
        59, 115, 166
stand-alone table 6, 46
State Inpatient Database (SID) 4–5, 47,
        49, 92
stepwise regression 169–170

straight-line network flow map 77,
    187–188, 193, 195
sub-community (network analysis) 124,
    126–127, 159
subnetwork 9, 124, 126, 142
supply-based thiessen approach 94

tertiary hospital market area 1
Thiessen polygon 94–97
threshold population (in the central
    place theory) 42
threshold population size 9, 68, 74,
    88–89, 92, 125, 151
topological distances 11, 13
trade areas 2, 8, 93
transit travel time matrix 19, 21
travel modes 17, 23–24, 28, 30, 98
travel-time-based proximal area 100–101
2SFCA *see* two-step floating catchment
    area (2SFCA) method
turn impedance 12
two-step floating catchment area
    (2SFCA) method 43–44

undirected network 155
undirected weighted network 66, 122
unimodal distribution 50
unitary elasticity 45–46, 156
unitary exponent (gravity model) 103
urban cluster 168
urban sphere of influence 2
urbanicity 49–51, 60, 166, 168
urbanized area 168
urbanization ratio 166, 168, 170
U.S. Postal Service 36

variation inflation factor 169
Voronoi polygon 94

wait time 37
web mapping service 37

XY To Line tool 73, 188, 193–194

ZIP-to-ZIP drive time matrix 32–33,
    37, 173